Yoga Complete

The All-in-One Yoga Guide – 40 Poses for Every Skillset

I0411945

Yoga Complete

The All-in-One Yoga Guide – 40 Poses for Every Skillset

By Robert Junior

© Copyright 2015 Robert Junior

Preface

First of all, let me tell you how happy I am for downloading my book. *"Yoga Complete: The All-in-One Yoga Guide – 40 Poses for Every Skillset"*.

This book is the sequel of my first book of the series "Yoga for Beginners: The Modern Guide Of Yoga Poses for Beginners To Practice Meditation And Yoga In Less Than 24 Hours". If you enjoyed my first book...well this one is going to blow your mind away.

In this new sequel I have included over 40 Yoga poses from beginner to intermediate and finally to advanced level - that is the logical sequence of the first yoga poses for beginners. Hopefully by now you have mastered these easy poses and you are ready for your next step in the wonderful world of yoga.

Take control today, and come with me for a life-changing journey through the beautiful world of transcendence and mental awareness.

Thanks again for downloading this book, I hope you enjoy it!

Table of Contents

Introduction

If you're reading this book, you're most likely not brand new at yoga. Never the less this book is a complete guide so it includes many poses from various levels of difficulty. About one fourth of poses in this book are for amateurs and the rest for intermediate to advanced level. Therefore, I will briefly outline what you most likely already know. Yoga is more than a form of exercise. It is a lifestyle that people choose due to the mental, emotional, and physical benefits.

Some of the physical benefits include:

- Increased muscle strength, tone, flexibility, and balance.
- Increased vitality, energy, metabolism and improved respiration.
- Weight loss.
- Improved cardio health.
- And protection from injury.

Mental benefits include:

- The ability to manage stress.
- Development of coping skills.
- Develop a better outlook on life.

Emotional benefits include:

- Increased self-esteem.
- Ability to remain calm.

Before you begin with yoga poses, let's take a look at some of the safety precautions you should take.

- Find an excellent, reputable instructor who is certified if you choose to practice within a classroom environment. They're knowledgeable about whether or not your body will be able to perform the poses they're displaying, and they should know what you can and cannot do if you have any type of injury or ailment.
- Do not treat yoga as a competition. This is a good way to get hurt while you're in a classroom or yoga environment because there are others out there who will be more advanced and flexible than you. If you push yourself too hard too fast, you risk injury.
- Be sure to stay within your limits. If you start to feel pain or severe discomfort, stop the pose immediately and go back to something easier.
- Warm-up before you begin. It's important to have your muscles loose and relaxed before you start twisting into poses. Cold muscles are more easily injured and less likely to be fluid enough to do intermediate poses. If you're comfortable with beginner poses, try doing a few of those before you slide into the intermediate poses.

Finally, what you'll need in order to practice the poses described within this book.

A quiet place. You'll want somewhere that you're not distracted because yoga is more than just physical, it's about the calmness of your mind.

A yoga mat or soft place outside. There's a possibility you may lose your balance with these poses, so having somewhere that you can get an easy grip and fall softly is a good idea.

A relaxed mental and physical state. Pretty self-explanatory, but you should be warm and loose from stretching and relaxed from a round of meditation before you begin.

Now that you're informed and prepared let's take a look at some Yoga techniques!

I have noted every Yoga pose with an indicative difficulty level system – 1 star being the easiest ones, to 5 stars for the most advanced ones - in case you want to escalate from the most basic ones to the most advanced.

Archer Pose (★★★★☆)

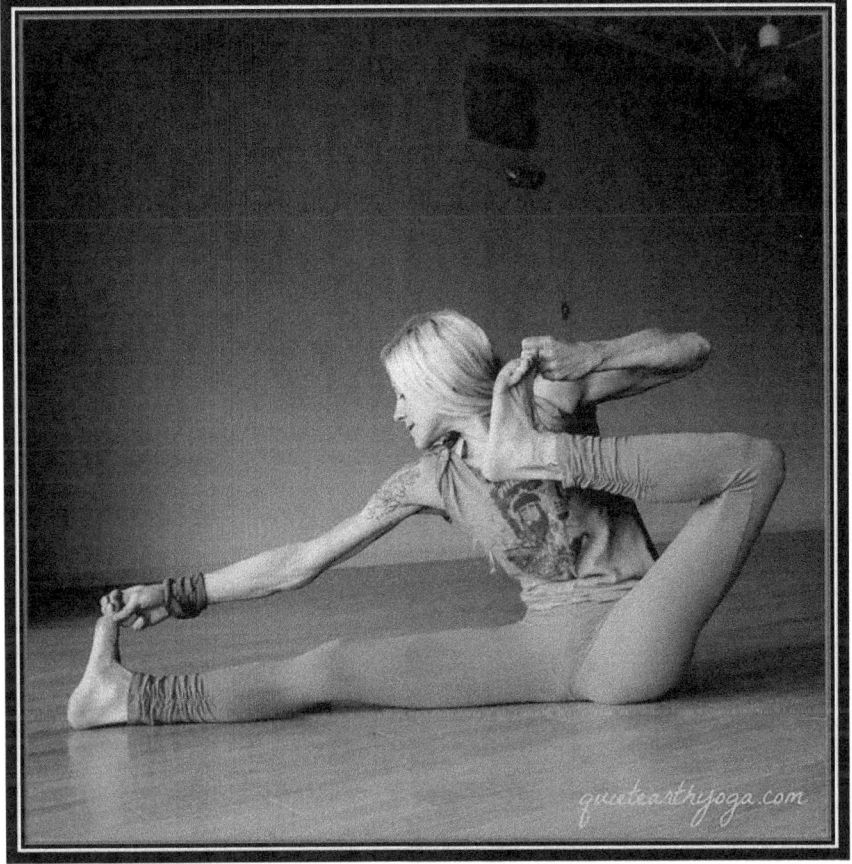

Photo courtesy of Amy at Flickr.com

The archer pose will strengthen your arms, abs, and back, and it will stretch those hamstrings as well as your calves.

1. To begin, sit in the staff position with your legs extended in front of you and your back straight. Reach forward and grab a hold of your toes and bend your knees gently if you have to in order to keep your back from rounding.

2. Exhale and use your right hand to pull your right foot close to your torso as you bend your knee. Keep your left arm and leg in their original positions. If you feel that this is enough, stay in this position.

3. If you feel you can go further, bring your right heel closer to your right ear and extend your lifted leg out as straight as you can.

4. To come out of the pose, exhale, and release your foot and extend it back to the floor.

5. Now do the other side!

Bird of Paradise (★★★★★)

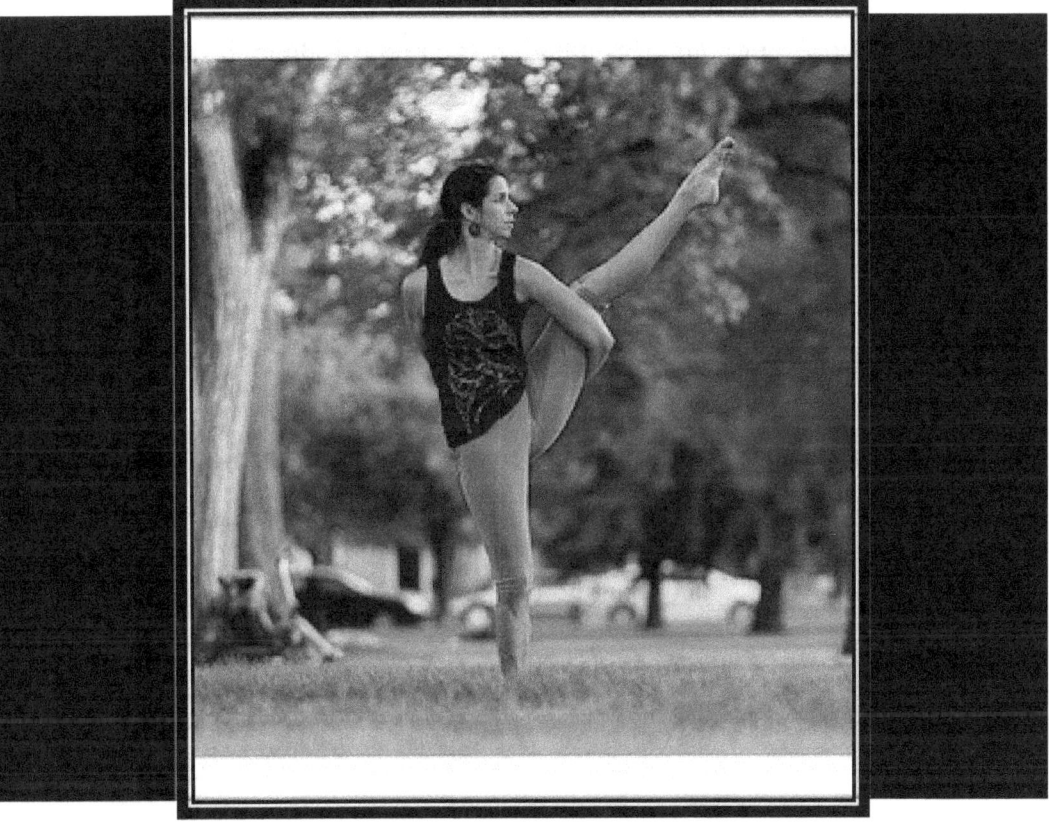

Photo courtesy of a4gpa at Flickr.com

The bird of paradise pose will strengthen your legs and stretch your inner thighs, hips, groin, shoulders and chest. It will also lengthen your spine. It's good for people who have a scattered mind, poor balance, and need more grace.

1. Begin in the mountain pose. Step your feet apart widely and turn your right leg out ninety degrees and your left leg in by forty-five degrees.

2. Raise your arms out to the sides at your shoulders and look to your right. Bend your right knee to ninety degrees and come into the virabhadrasana II pose.

3. Now, put your right hand on the floor inside your right foot with your fingertips pointed the same direction as your toes. Place your right sin and your right arm together. Reach your left arm up and extend it overhead to the right with your palm facing down.

4. Lower your left arm behind you and bend the elbow so that you can put your left palm on your right thigh. Interlace your hands behind you.

5. Now, gaze at the floor and bend your right knee and lift your right leg. Keep the knee bent. Straighten your left leg in order to stand. Straighten that right leg and hold for two breaths. Slowly release and do the other side.

Boat (★★☆☆☆)

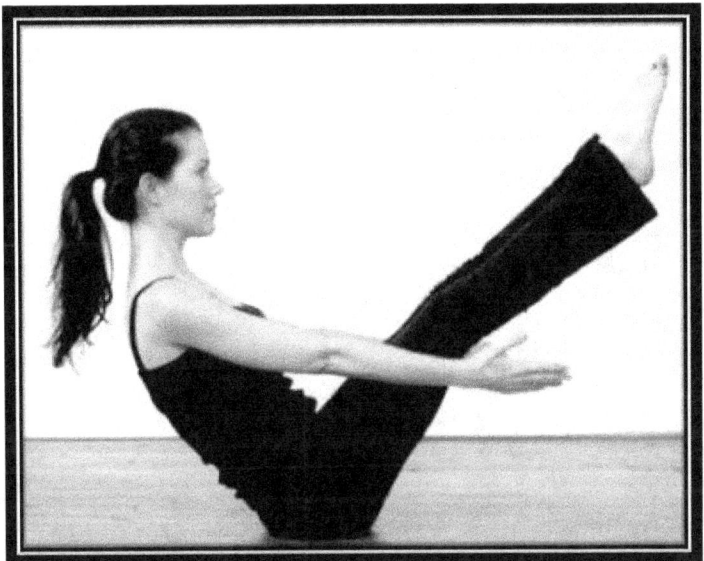

Photo courtesy of tongerandy at photobucket.com

The boat position is great to use to strengthen your abs, back and thighs. It helps with a weak core, balance, focus, self-confidence, and bloating.

1. To begin, sit on the floor and keep your knees bent but your feet flat on the floor. Grab your legs under your thighs.
2. Lean back a little and lift your feet off the floor. Keep them pressed together and lift until your shins are parallel to the floor.
3. Extend your arms straight at shoulder height with your palms facing each other.
4. Straighten your legs until you've formed a 'v' shape and balance on your glutes, not your lower back.
5. Hold this position for three to five breaths and then gently lower your shins first, and your hands on your thighs.

Bound Angle (★☆☆☆☆)

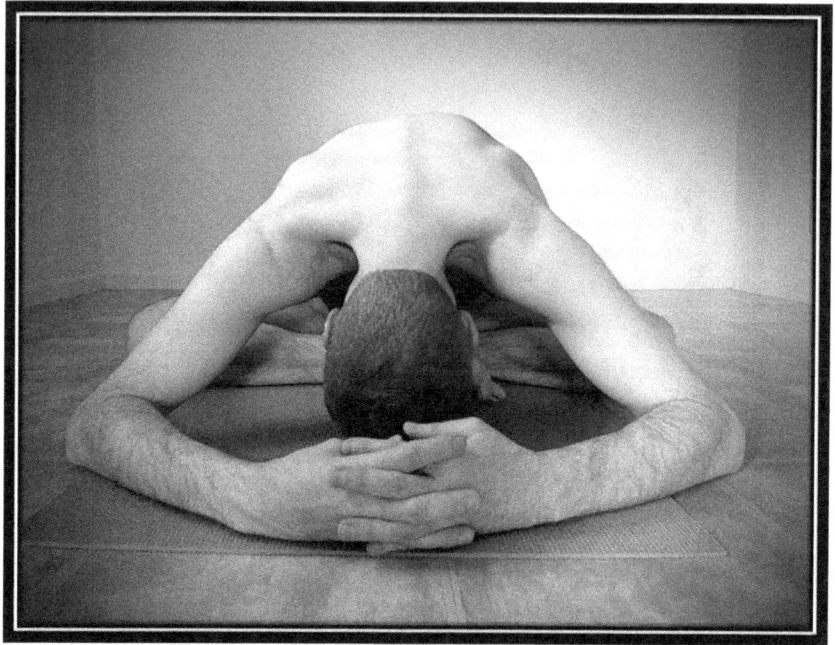

Photo courtesy of Nicholas A. Tonelli at Flickr.com

While it may not look difficult at first, you'll be surprised by how hard it is to get into this position. However, once you do, you'll realize that it's stretching your hips, thighs, groin, and lengthening your spine. This position has been known to help with anxiety, fatigue, and sciatica.

1. Come to a sitting position with your soles of your feet touching. Take hold of your big toes with your first and two fingers and thumb. Bring your heels close to your groin area.

2. Lower your knees to the floor and stretch your spine tall and straight. Now, gently bend forward until you reach the limit of your stretch. Remember, do not go too far!

3. If you feel you can, you may lower your forehead to the floor and hold the position for ten seconds.

Bow (★★★☆☆)

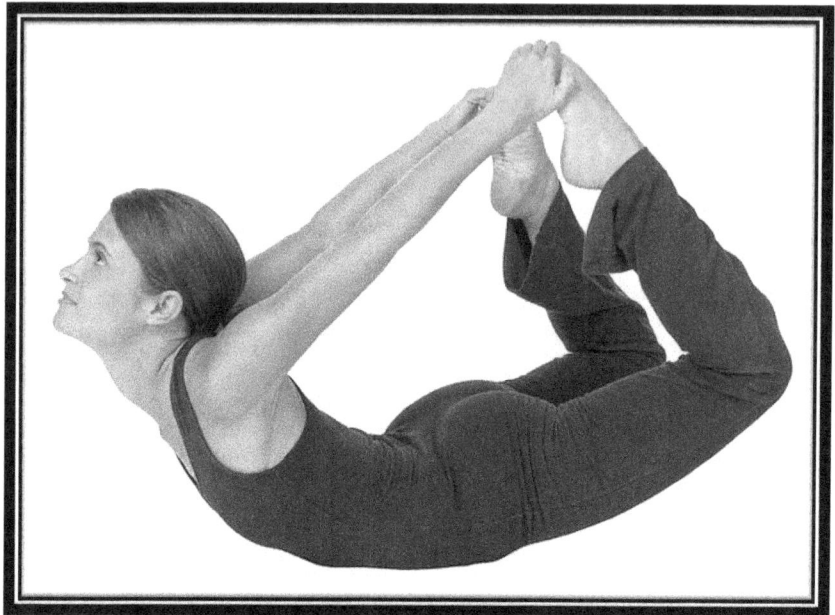

Photo courtesy of IDIA 642 Images at Flickr.com

The bow is a great move that will stretch out your entire body and strengthen your core as well as keep your spine flexible. It helps with those who are feeling fatigued.

1. Lay down on the floor front down. Lift your chest and rest your forearms parallel to each other in front of you. Come into the sphinx pose.
2. Bend your right leg and reach back to grab your right ankle with your right hand. Do the same with your left.
3. Keep your feet flexed and raise your chest off the floor and lift both of your knees. Breathe deeply and hold for five seconds.

4. To come out of the pose, gently let go of your ankles and slide your legs down. Then relax your arms and your front and lie down for a few seconds.

Br

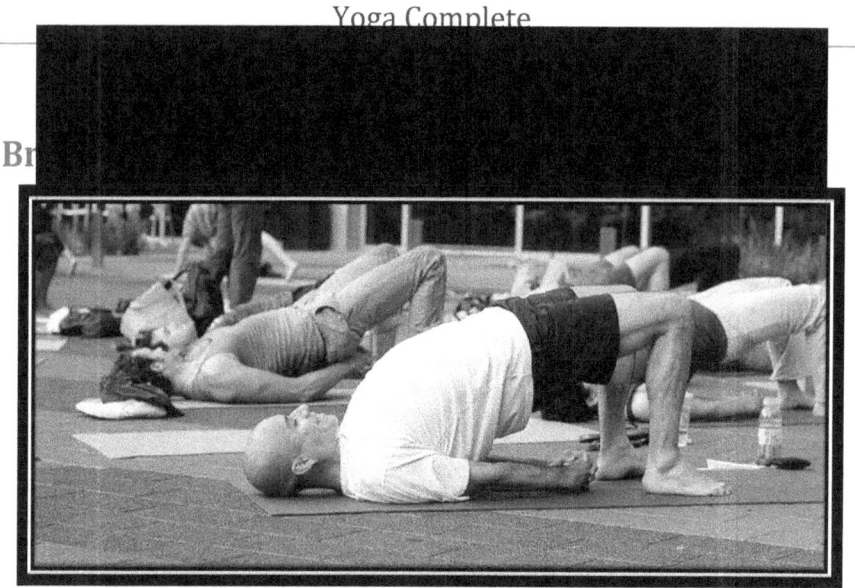

Photo courtesy of adrian Valenzuela at Flickr.com

The bridge position is excellent for your back, thighs, glutes chest, hips, quads, and your spine. It helps with intestinal function as well as anxiety and fatigue.

1. Lie down on your back and put your feet flat on the floor. Place your arms beside you with your palms down.
2. Start by lifting your torso up off the ground vertebrae by vertebrae until all of your weight is on your shoulders.
3. Now interlace your hands beneath and behind you and draw your glutes toward your knees.
4. Hold for five seconds and separate your arms slowly to slide out of the position.

Ca

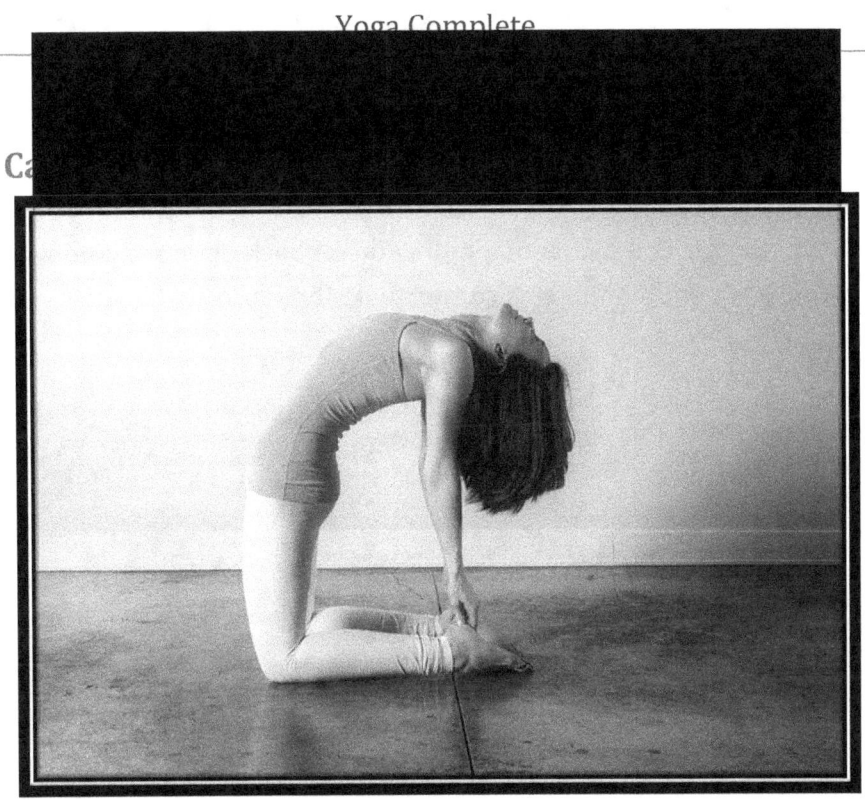

Photo courtesy of Jon Fife at Flickr.com

The camel pose may seem easy to perform, but it's a good workout for your chest, abs, groin, and thighs. This position is recommended for those who suffer from depression and poor posture.

1. Kneel on the floor with your hips directly above your knees. Your shoulders should be above your hips so you are sitting straight.
2. Place your palms on the small of your back and have your fingertips facing up. If you are not comfortable, you can put your fingertips facing the ground, too.
3. Inhale and lengthen your spine. Expand your chest and slowly lower yourself backward until you are able to grip your ankles. Try to form a square.

4. Hold this position as you breathe deeply for five seconds. To come out of the post, you can slowly slide backward until you're touching the floor and slide your legs out from under you, or you can gently pull yourself back up into a kneeling position. Whatever is comfortable for you.

Chair Pose (★★☆☆☆)

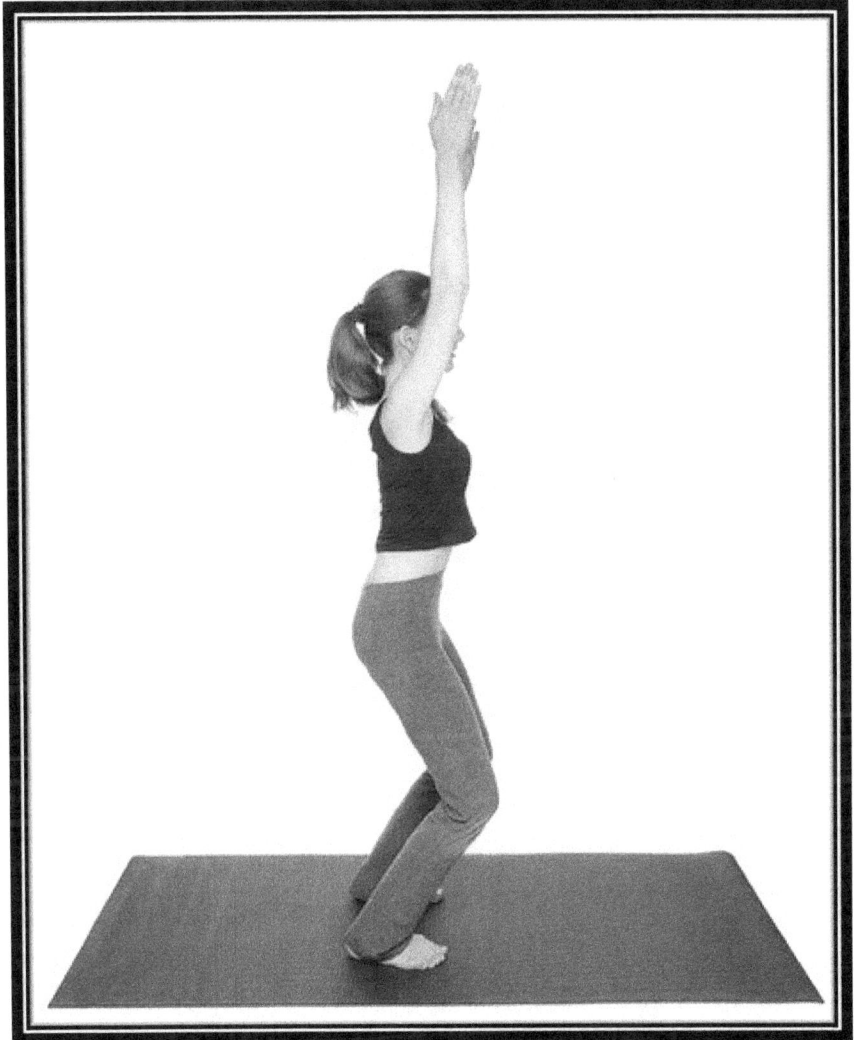

Photo courtesy of dgilder at Flickr.com

The chair pose is another deceivingly simple looking pose that is actually rather difficult considering it uses your upper back strength, glutes, thighs, calves, and ankles. This posture is excellent for posture, timidity, and endurance.

1. Get into a standing position and keep your arms at your side, or the mountain position.
2. Bend your knees deeply and shift your weight back onto your heels. Squeeze your inner thighs together.
3. Straighten your arms and raise them overhead. Bring your back into a slight bend as if you were going to sit in a chair, and hold that position.
4. Hold for ten breaths at the very least.

C

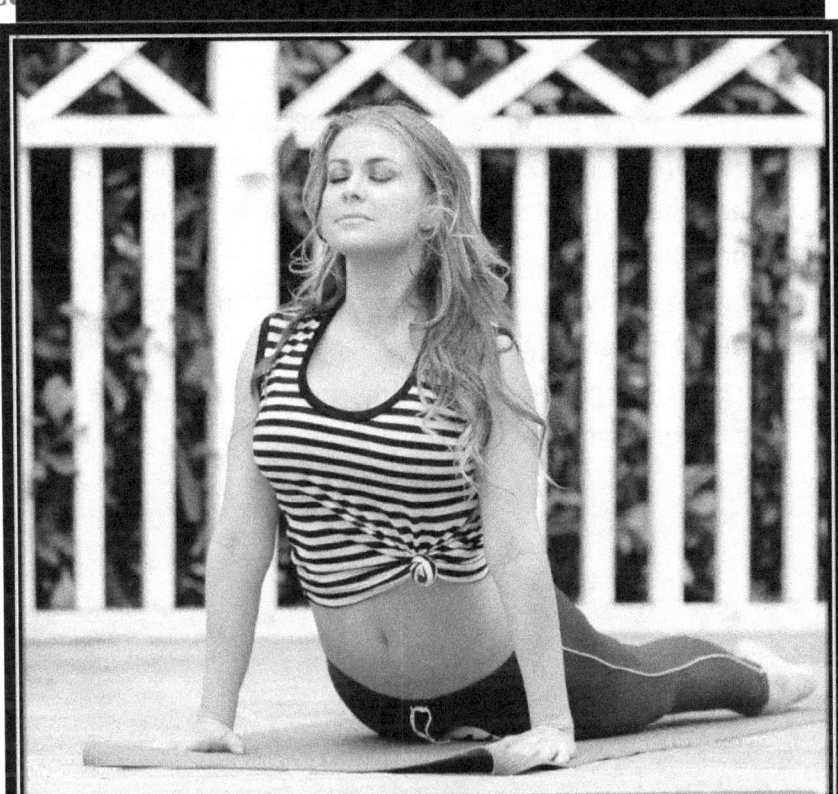

Photo courtesy of manujadon007 at photobucket.com

The full cobra position is a lot more difficult to perform because it works your thighs, glutes, hamstrings, abs, back, and your chest all at the same time. It looks pretty easy, but it's actually strenuous. This pose is excellent for those who suffer from poor posture, depression, low energy and lower back discomfort.

1. Lay down on the floor with your front on the floor. Press your toes and forehead to the floor gently. Rest your palms

on either side of your chest and your finger pointing forward.

2. Lift your shoulders and chest off the floor using your palms and your arms to lift upward.

3. Keep your chest up and extend all the way up until your arms are straight. Do not allow the elbow to bend outward, keep them straight. This can cause tennis elbow if not done correctly.

4. Now make sure your hips are lifted off the ground too and your glutes are tight.

5. Breathe deeply for five breaths and gently lower back down to the ground.

Cobra Modified (★★☆☆☆)

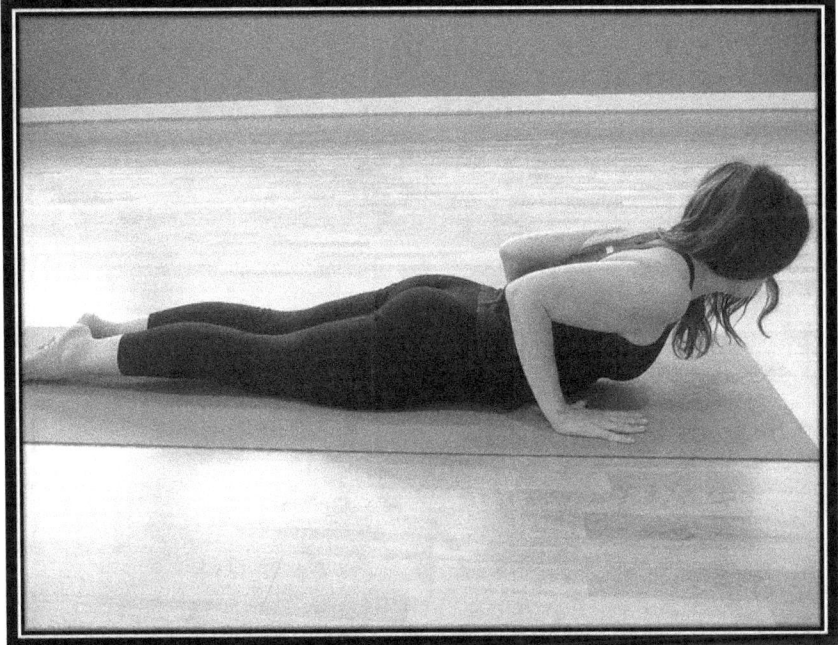

Photo courtesy of yogamama at Flickr.com

The modified cobra is a little easier to perform but still helps strengthen your back, glutes, hamstrings, chest, and abs. It's also great for posture, your back, depression, and fatigue.

1. Lay face down on the floor and press your toes and forehead to the floor.
2. Rest your palm on either side of your chest and keep your elbows bent.
3. Now press toward the floor lightly and come up until your upper arms are parallel to the floor. Bring your palms off the floor a moment and then place them back down gently.

Cow Face (★★★★☆)

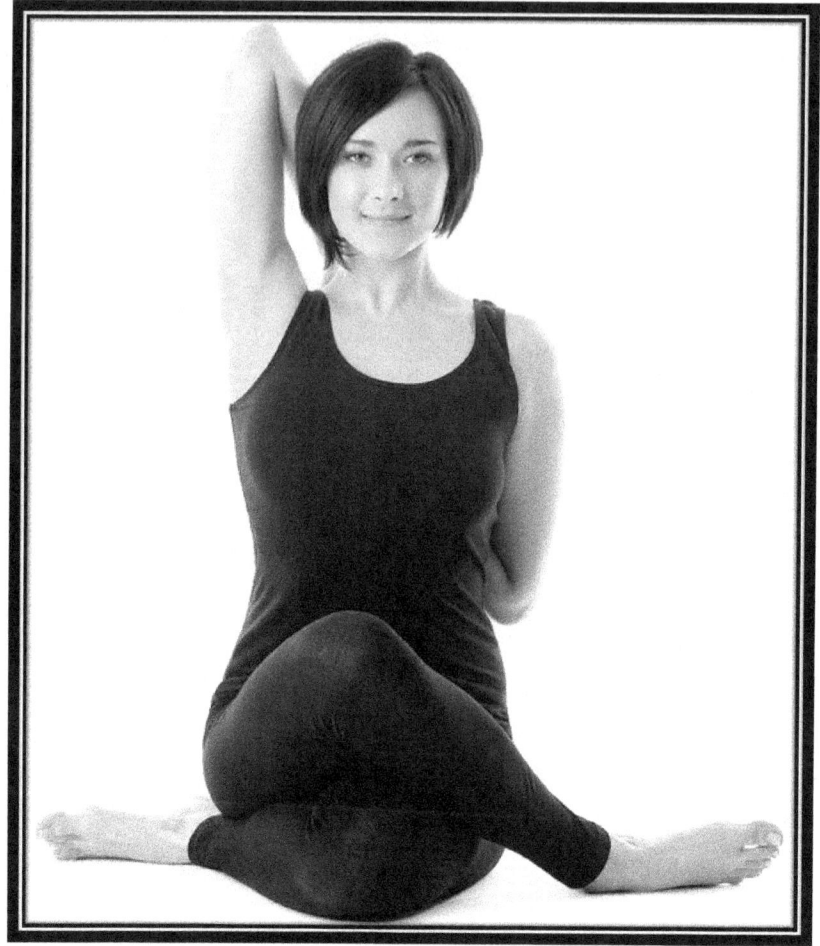

Photo courtesy of Melanie Sarta at Flickr.com

The cow face position is great for your shoulders, chest, armpits, hips, and ankles. It's for poor posture and tight shoulders.

1. Sit with your legs straight out in front of you.

2. Bend your right leg and cross it over your left. Now bend your left leg in and stack your knees with your left foot next to your right hip.

3. Now reach behind you with your left hand over your left shoulder and your right hand behind your back. Clasp your hands together and hold the position for five breaths. Switch your legs and your arms and do the other side.

4. If you want to get crazy, bend forward while doing this for an extra stretch, but only if you're comfortable with the first position!

Crescent Lunge (★★★☆☆)

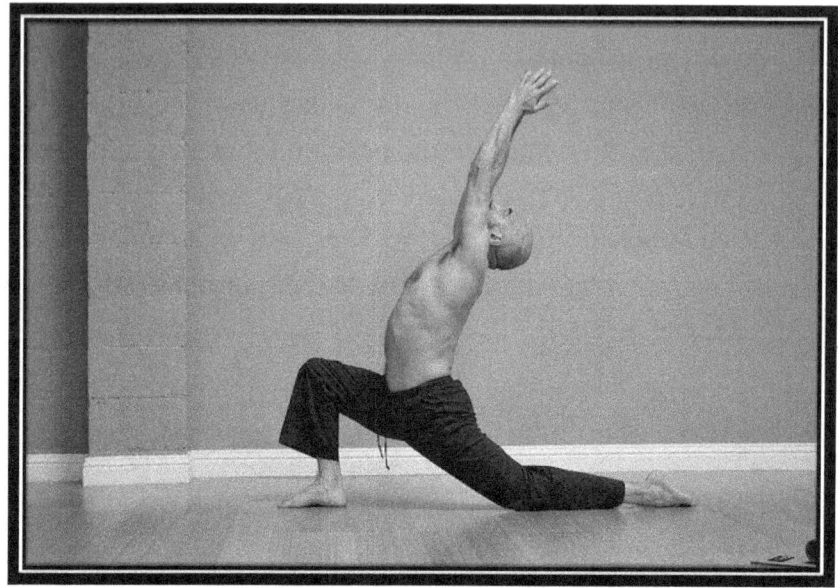

Photo courtesy of Clive Beavis at Fickr.com

The crescent lunge is excellent for your legs, hips, and balance.

1. Being in downward facing dog.
2. Step your right foot between your hands and lower your hips. Lower your left knee to the floor and untuck your toes. Press the top of your left foot into the floor.
3. Bring your arms up and overhead and touch your palms together. Bend back gently and clasp your hands. Deepen the backbend and keep your abs tight. Then return to an upright position.
4. Hold for five breaths and then gently slide out of the pose, back into downward facing dog.

Cross-Legged Forward Bend (★★★☆☆)

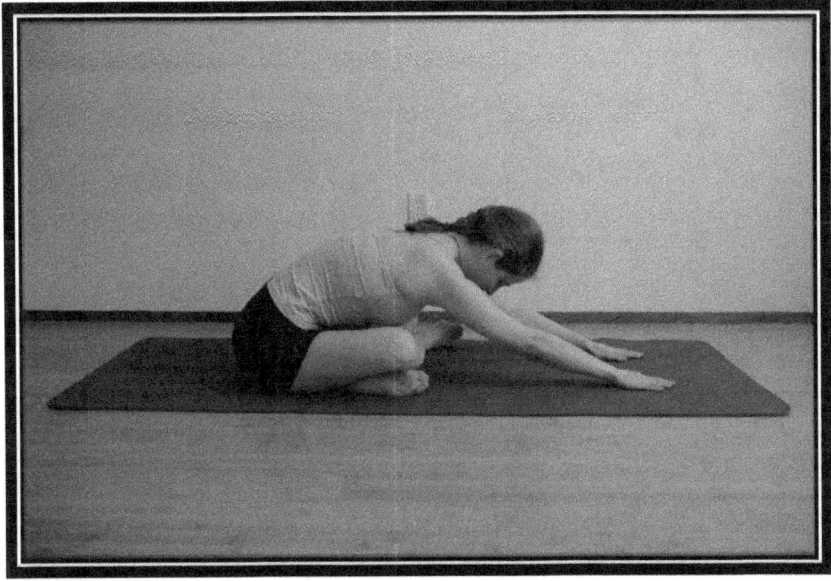

Photo courtesy of Tiffany Berry at Flickr.com

This pose is great for your hips, back shoulders, thighs, and your spine. Most people use this pose for meditation and stress.

1. Sit in a cross-legged position. Inhale and exhale deeply three times and then place your hands on the floor in front of you. Lift your hips as you do so.
2. Now bend over your legs gently as far as you can go and rest there for another three breaths, or as long as you're comfortable.
3. Sit up gently, inhaling and exhaling three times.
4. You can stay in this pose as long as you wish while you meditate.

Crow (★★★★★)

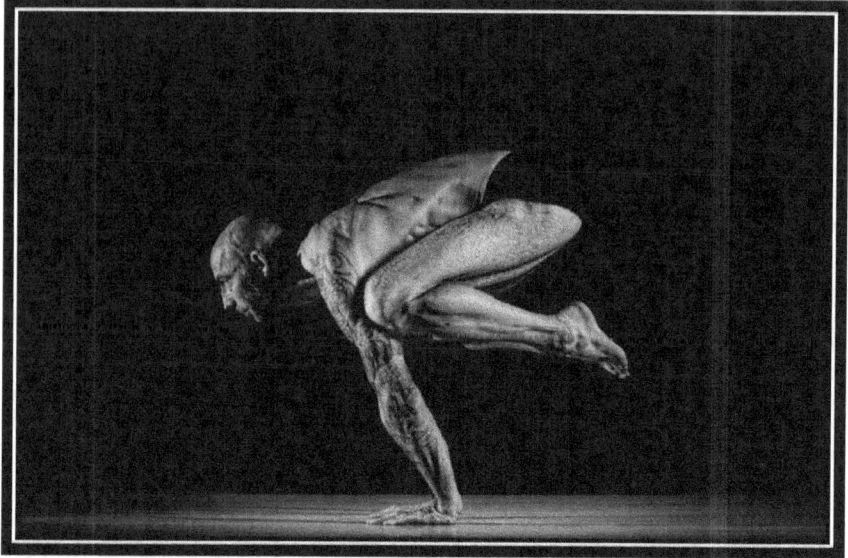

Photo courtesy of Christian Eberle at Flickr.com

Deceptively simple looking, the crow is great for strengthening your arms, shoulders, chest, abs and back. It's good to use if you suffer from a weak back, bad posture, coordination, and focus.

1. Begin in a deep squat, also known as malasana.
2. Put your hands on the floor in front of you, they should line up with your shoulders. Come up onto your tiptoes and walk your feet closer to your hands. Shift your weight forward into your hands and bring your knees up onto your elbows.
3. You may not be able to get your knees up to your elbows on the first few tries, so keep them on your elbows if you must instead.
4. Hold this position for three breaths and then gently slide out of it the way you got into it.

Da

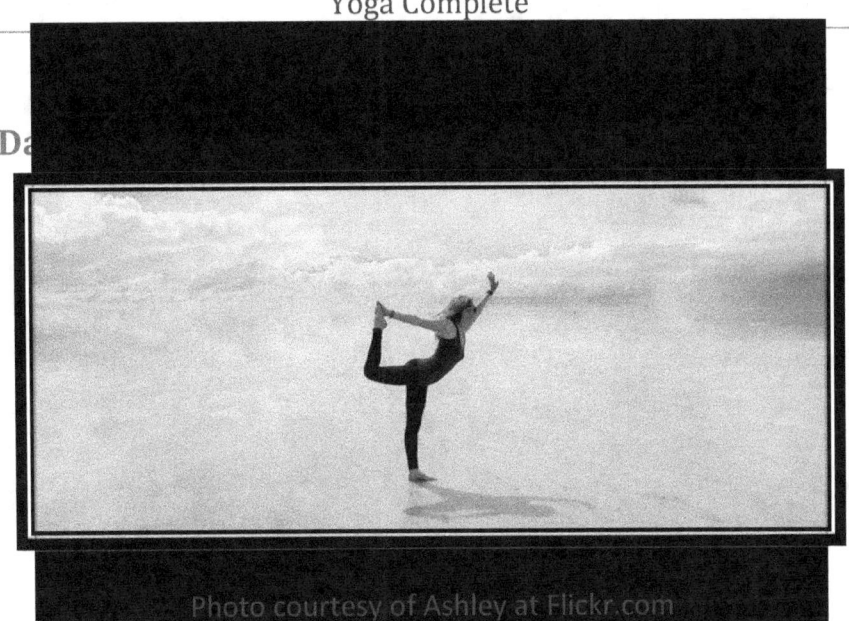

Photo courtesy of Ashley at Flickr.com

The dancer pose is most likely one of the most infamous yoga poses. It's great for your ankles, legs, thighs, groin, hips, abs, chest, shoulders and spine. People perform this pose to help with their balance, poise, energy levels, and stamina.

1. Stand in the mountain pose. Keep your feet in line with your hips and your hands by your sides.
2. Bend your right knee and reach back. Lift your right leg up and grasp your right ankle with your right hand. Try to come up as far as possible.
3. To keep your balance, reach your left hand out with your fingers pointed directly out and stay parallel with the ground.
4. Hold the position for five breaths and then switch to the other side.

Double Big Toe Hold (★★★☆☆)

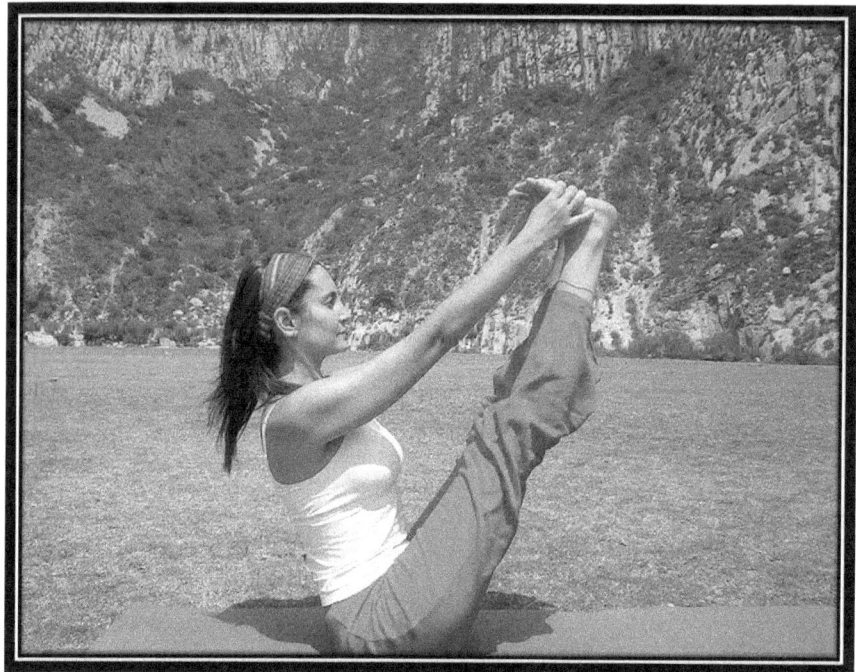

Photo courtesy of luisdemiguel at Flickr.com

The key to this position is balance. It helps with strengthening your core, legs, back, hamstrings, calves, and your spine. People use this pose to help with their balance, poise, and self-confidence.

1. Sit on the floor with your knees bent and your feet flat on the floor. Your hands should be on your knees.
2. Now, gently raise your legs in the air, keeping them parallel with one another. Grasp your big toes with both hands, using your two first fingers and your thumb to do so. Form a 'v' shape and hold for as long as comfortable.
3. Gently let go of your toes and slide out of the position when you're finished.

Down-Dog-To-Plank Sequence (★☆☆☆☆)

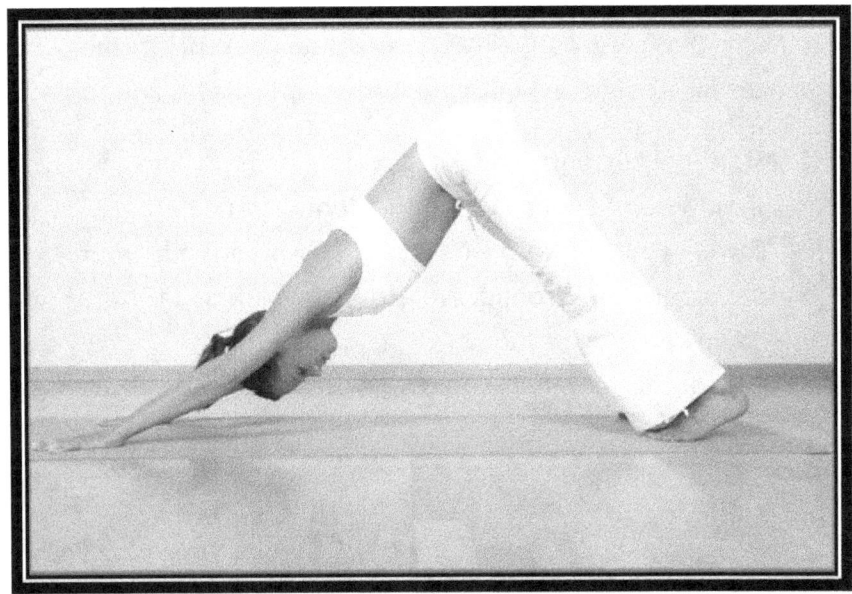

Photo courtesy of yogagirl1_bucket at photobucket.com

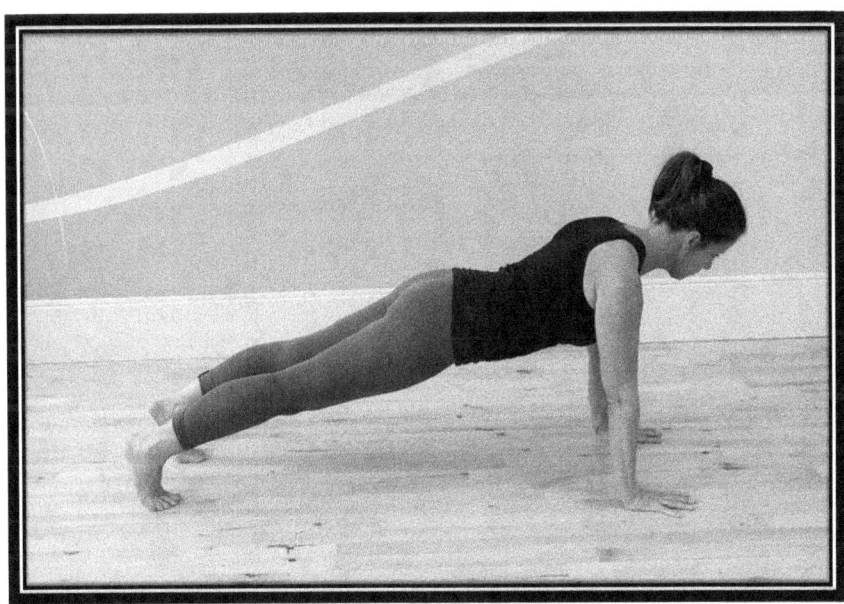

Photo courtesy of yogamama at Flickr.com

If you're looking for a sequence that will get your cardio going and help with your core as well as your back, look no further. This sequence will strengthen your core, arms, hips, thighs, and spine.

1. Start on all fours and keep your hands in line with your shoulders and your toes on the floor.
2. Lower yourself into the plank position with your body parallel to the ground. Now raise your hips in the air into downward dog position.
3. Repeat this ten times and take a break.

Eagle (★★★★★)

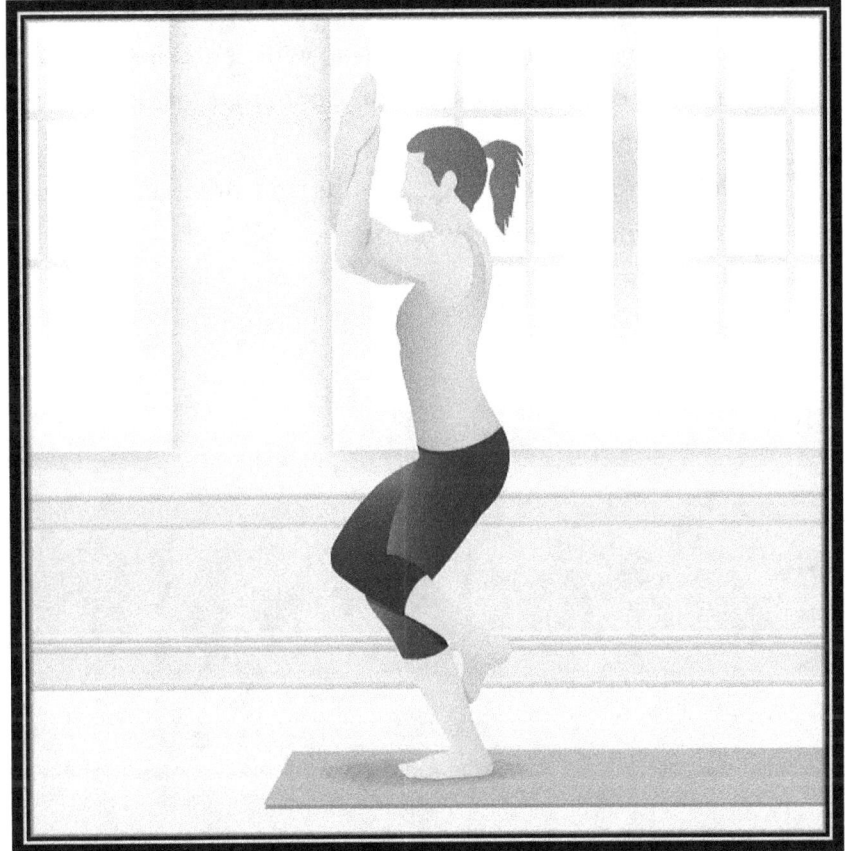

Photo courtesy of Gaurav Mishra at Flickr.com

The eagle position is great for strengthening your ankles, knees, thighs, abs, and stretching your upper back. People perform it to help with their self-confidence, as well as their poise and legs.

1. Begin in the mountain pose with your feet in line with your shoulders and your arms to your sides.
2. Raise your arms out to be parallel with the ground and your palms should be facing down. Cross your arms in front of

you at the elbows with your left elbow on top. Bend your elbows and bring the palms together.

3. Lift your right foot and make your leg parallel with the ground. Cross your right leg over your left thigh and hook your toes behind your left calf. Bend your left knee, lower your hips, and squat.

4. Hold this for three to five breaths and then gently release your left and untwist your arms.

5. Switch sides.

Extended Big Toe Hold (★★★★☆)

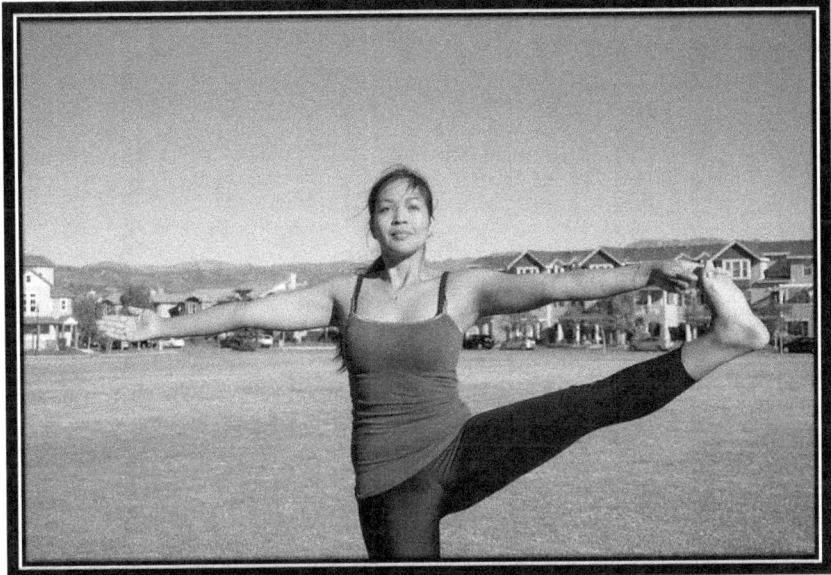

Photo courtesy of 805 Promo at Flickr.com

The extended toe hold is great for balance and poise. It stretches your legs, ankles, knees, abs, back and hamstrings.

1. Come to the mountain pose with your arms at your sides. Bring your right foot up your left leg slowly and extend your right arm so that it's parallel to the ground.
2. Extend your right leg so that it is parallel to the ground and grasp your right toe with your right hand using the first two fingers and your thumb.
3. Hold for five breaths and then release gently.
4. Switch sides.

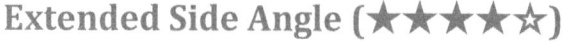

Extended Side Angle (★★★★☆)

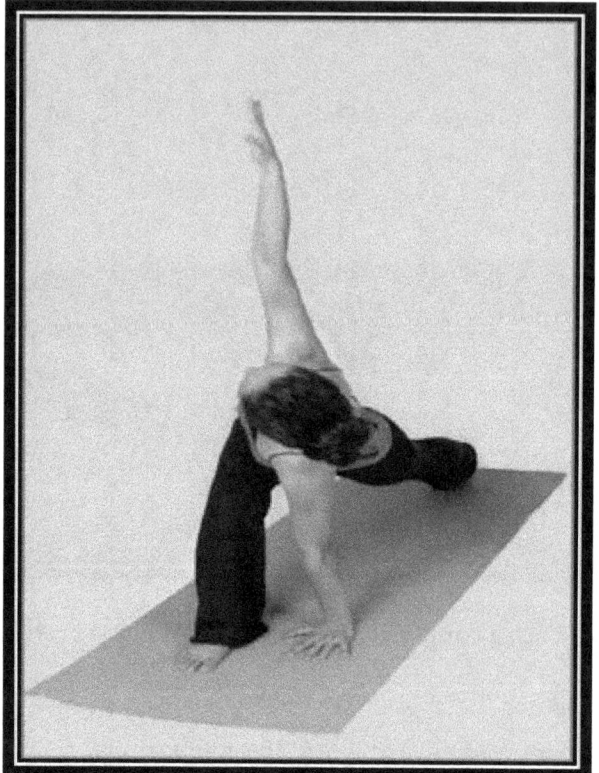

Photo courtesy of bryankestteacherstraining at photobucket.com

The extended side angle is excellent for strengthening your ankles, legs, core, upper arms, legs, hips, chest, and shoulders. People perform the pose for endurance, breathing, focus, their sciatica, and digestion.

1. Begin by standing in warrior pose II, found <u>here</u>.
2. Lower your left hand to the floor inside of your left foot and reach your right arm up.
3. Rotate your right arm by using our shoulder blade and extend your body into one long line from the outside of your

right foot through the fingertips of your right hand, as shown.

4. Hold for five breaths and then gently twist your core so that you're straight and slide your leg back to be parallel with the ground.

5. Switch sides.

Firefly (★★★★★)

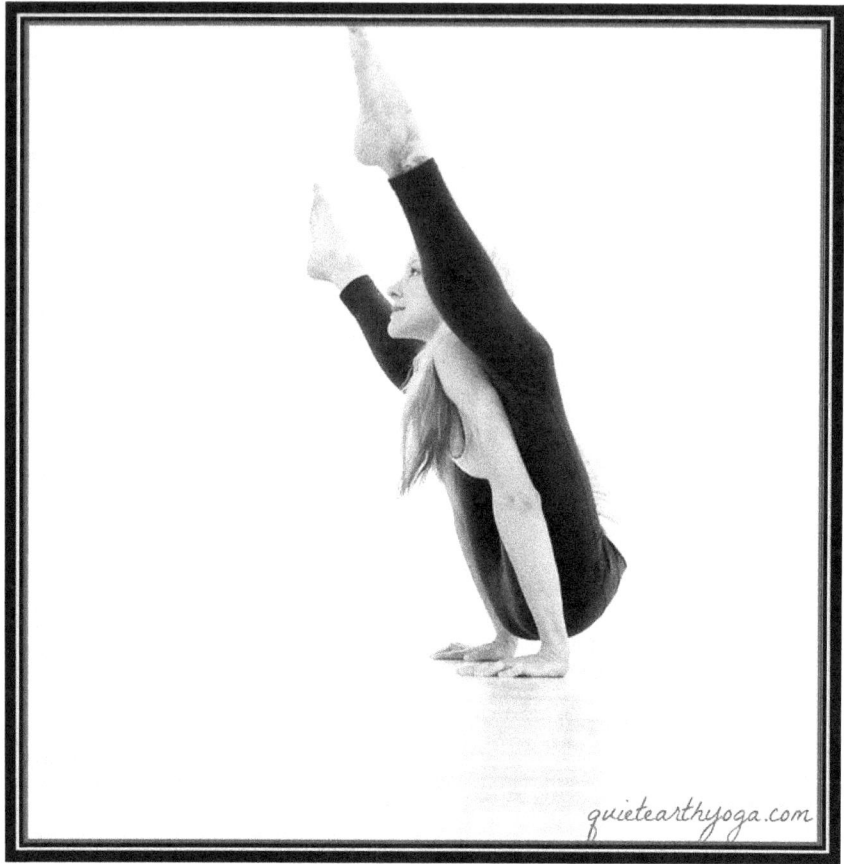

Photo courtesy of Amy at Flickr.com

The firefly pose is excellent for strengthening your arms, shoulders, abs, wrists, and hamstrings.

1. Start in a wide-legged squat and your hands in front of you on the floor.
2. Wrap your hands behind and around your feet and reach your shoulders under your knees.
3. Lift your feet and put your weight onto your hands.

4. Hold for three breaths and gently slide your legs out of the position, slowly.

Fish (★★☆☆☆)

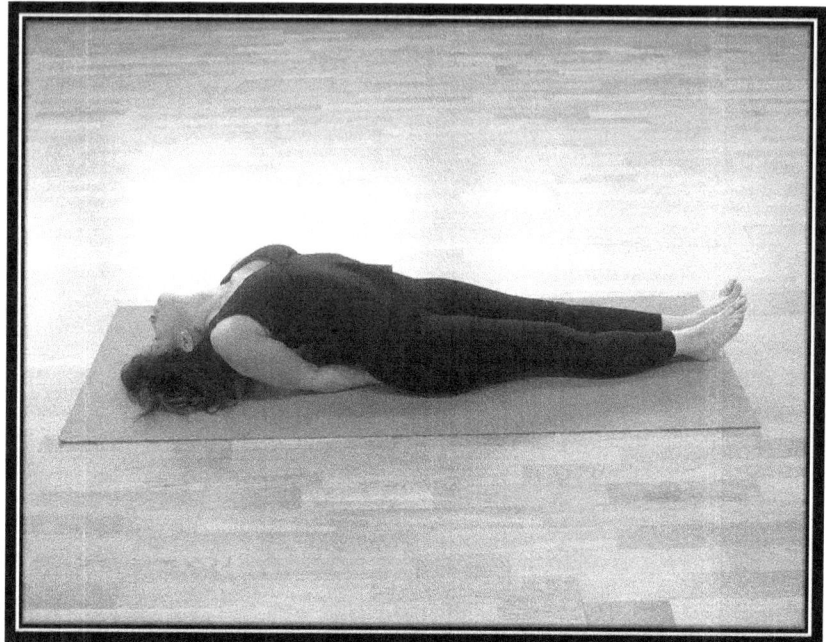

Photo courtesy of yogamama at Flickr.com

Another deceptively easy looking yoga position, but should only be performed by intermediate level yogis. The fish position is great for your chest, neck, hips, and upper back.

1. Lie on the floor on your back and keep your toes pointed skyward. Your arms should be alongside your body.
2. Now, place your palms on the floor and press your elbows into the floor. Arch your upper back and try to reach your heart toward the ceiling.
3. Pull your shoulders blade together and lift your chin.
4. Lean to the left and bring our right arm under your glutes and to the same for the other side. Hold for five breaths and gently slide out of the position.

Forearm Balance (★★★★☆)

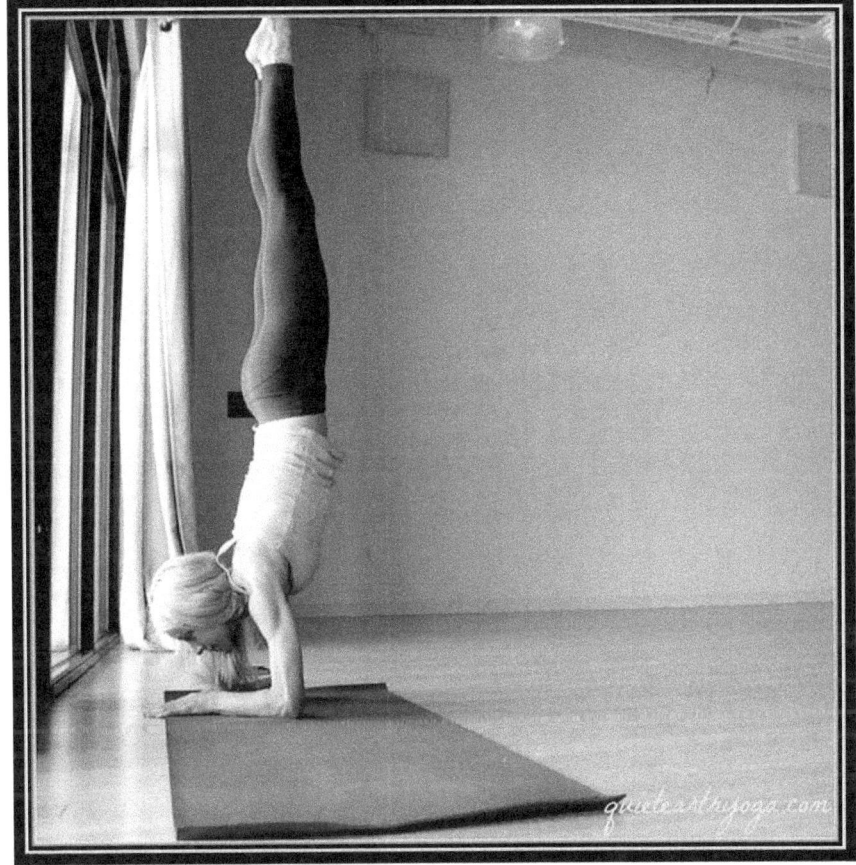

Photo courtesy of Amy at Flickr.com

The forearm balance is excellent for strengthening your core, arms, shoulders, back and chest. People use this for anxiety, fear, bad habits, and change of perspective.

1. Kneel with your behind resting on your heels. Place your forearms on the floor in front of you and keep them shoulder width apart.
2. Straighten your legs into dolphin pose.

3. Now lift your left foot toward the ceiling and lift your right leg up next. Squeeze your legs together and point your toes. Hold for two breaths and gently slide out of the position.

Frog (★★★☆☆)

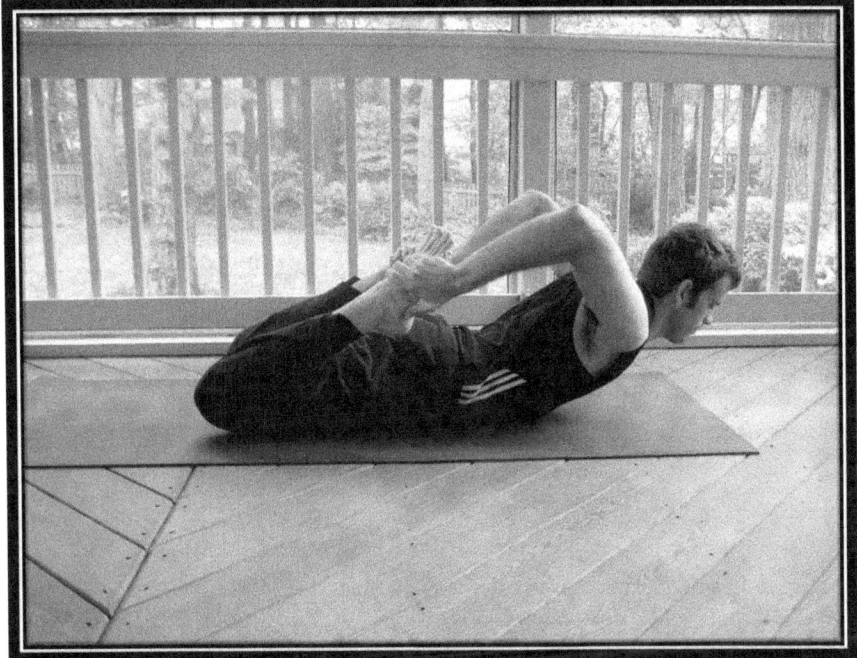

Photo courtesy of Chris at Flickr.com

The frog position strongly resembles the bow position and is also great for your thighs, hips and groin. People use this for digestion problems and knee pain.

1. Begin by getting on all fours and keep your knees at a wide stance. Lean forward as you lower your core to the floor.
2. Now rest your forearms on the floor and keep your torso above the floor.
3. Lower your torso until your body is on the floor and reach back to grasp your ankles.
4. Hold the position for four breaths and then release.

Half Moon (★☆☆☆☆)

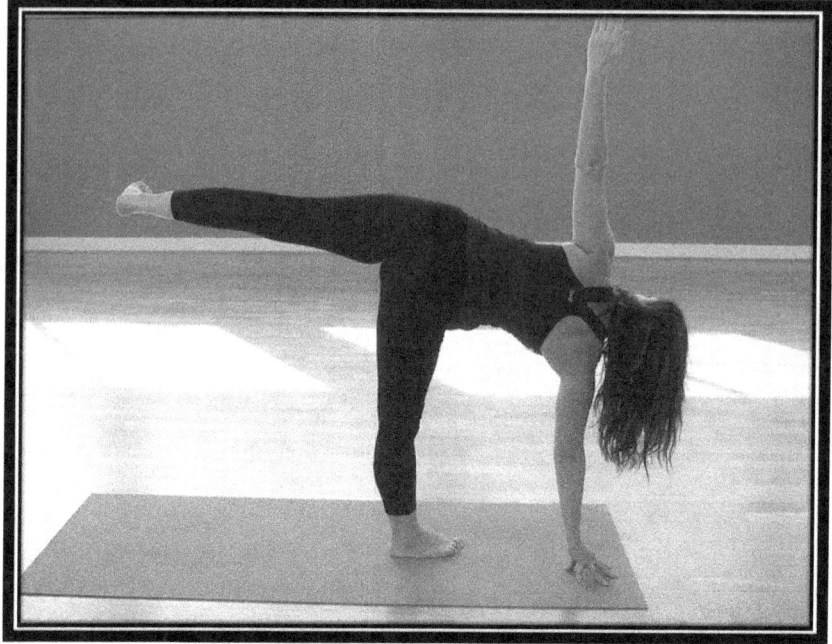

Photo courtesy of yogamama at Flickr.com

The half-moon position is great for your back, abs, knees, buttocks and hips. Yogis use it for balance endurance, self-confidence, and a scattered mind.

1. Begin in the triangle pose and keep your right leg in front.
2. Lower your left hand to your hip and put your right fingertips on the floor.
3. Lift your right leg into the air and straighten it.
4. Lift your right arm into the air and reach toward the sky.
5. Hold the position for five breaths and switch sides.

Handstand (★★★★☆)

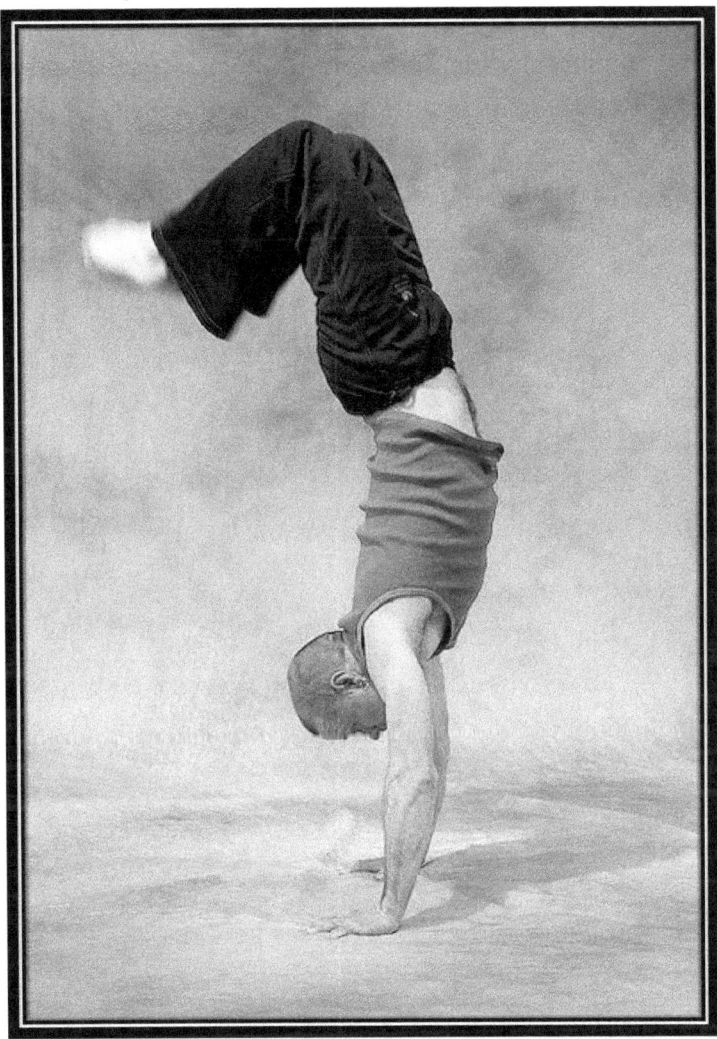

Photo courtesy of Patty Townsend at Flickr.com

A move that requires discipline and amazing balance, the handstand is not one that you want to try pulling off when you're a beginner. You can easily overcompensate and topple. This move is excellent for your shoulders, arms, wrists, core, legs, abs, and spine.

1. Place your hands on the floor in front of you and come into a downward facing dog pose.

2. Now do a few hops with each foot to get into position. When you're ready, hop up so that your feet are pointing to the ceiling, your head is hanging between your arms, and your arms are straight.

3. Hold the position for ten seconds and then release. You can rotate your hips if you're comfortable.

Happy Baby (★★★☆☆)

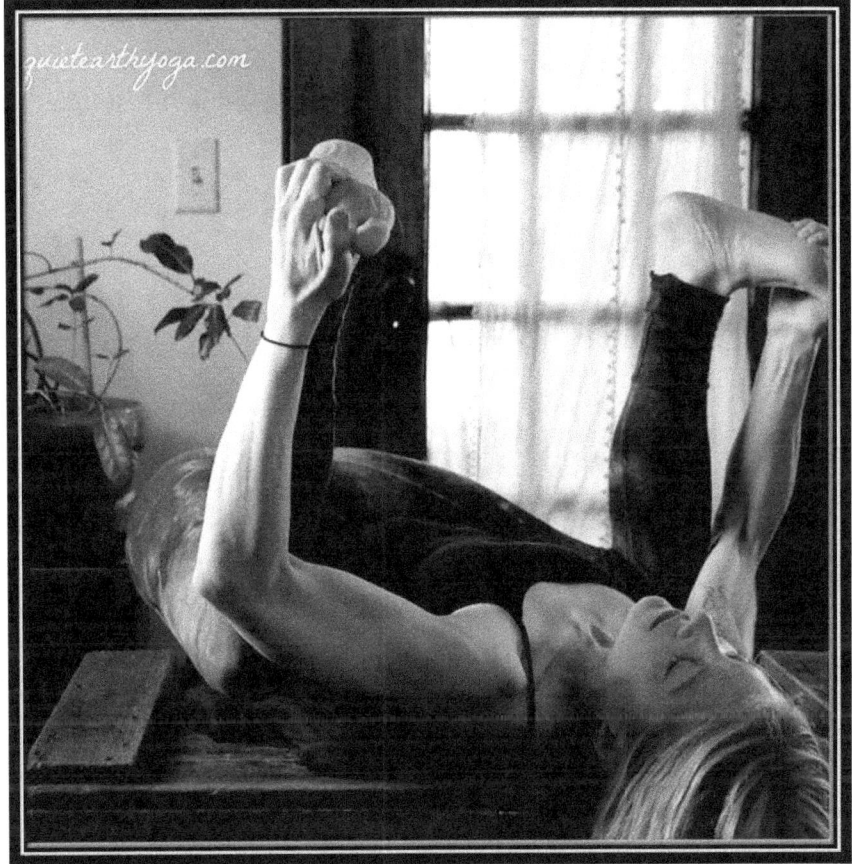

Photo courtesy of Amy at Flickr.com

The happy baby position is great for your inner thighs, groin, knees, and lower back. It helps with lower back discomfort and tight hips.

1. Lie down on your back and bring your knees up into a bent position. Keep your feet flat on the floor and your palms should be facing up.

2. Now bend your knees to your chest and separate them to the sides. Hold your shins or your toes with your fingers and bring your thighs down until they're parallel with the floor.
3. You should be able to bring your thighs down next to your torso, but don't stretch too far if you're not comfortable.
4. Hold for five breaths and then release.

Headstand (★★★★★)

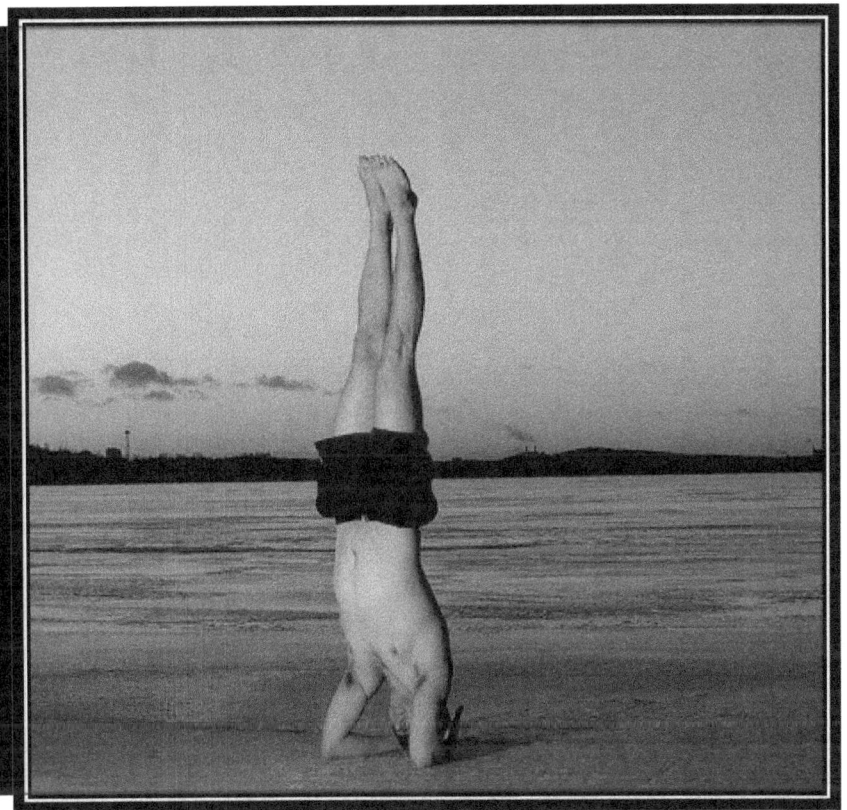

Photo courtesy of Sami Taipale at Flickr.com

The headstand requires a little less balance than the handstand, but it's still pretty difficult to perform when you're an adult. This is also great for your core, legs, spine, and arms.

1. Start with downward facing dog.
2. Move into dolphin pose and lower your forearms to the floor. Interlace your fingers together so that your arms form a triangle.

3. Now gently raise your legs above you, this may take a few tries, and hold for ten seconds. Keep your core tight and your legs tight.

4. Slide out of the pose gently and be careful not to fall.

Locust (★★★★☆)

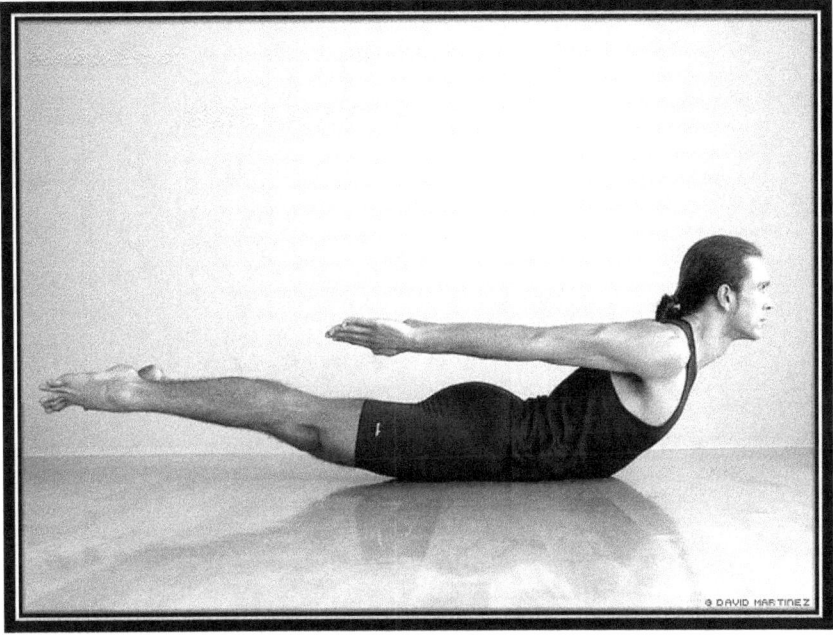

Photo courtesy of On Being at Flickr.com

It looks easy and pretty streamlined, but the locust pose is hard on your core and thigh muscles. It strengthens your back, buttocks, chest, shoulders, spine and helps with back pain as well as posture.

1. Lie face down on the floor and keep your arms alongside you with your palms facing up.
2. Bring your chest off the floor and keep your chin parallel to the ground.
3. Raise your arms to your chest and keep them parallel to the ground. Now raise your legs off the floor and keep your feet together.
4. Inhale and exhale a few times with your core muscles tightened and your buttocks tense.

5. Then slowly release.

Locust Variation (★★★★☆)

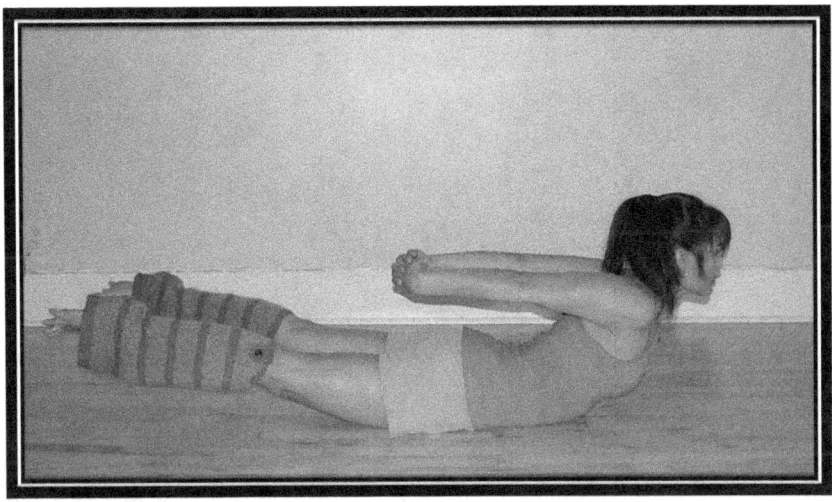

Photo courtesy of Elsie Escobar at Flickr.com

If you're comfortable with the first variation of the locust pose, try this one.

1. Come into the locust pose mentioned earlier, but place your arms behind your back and interlace your fingers together. This will stretch your shoulder blades and your chest.

Monkey (★★★★★)

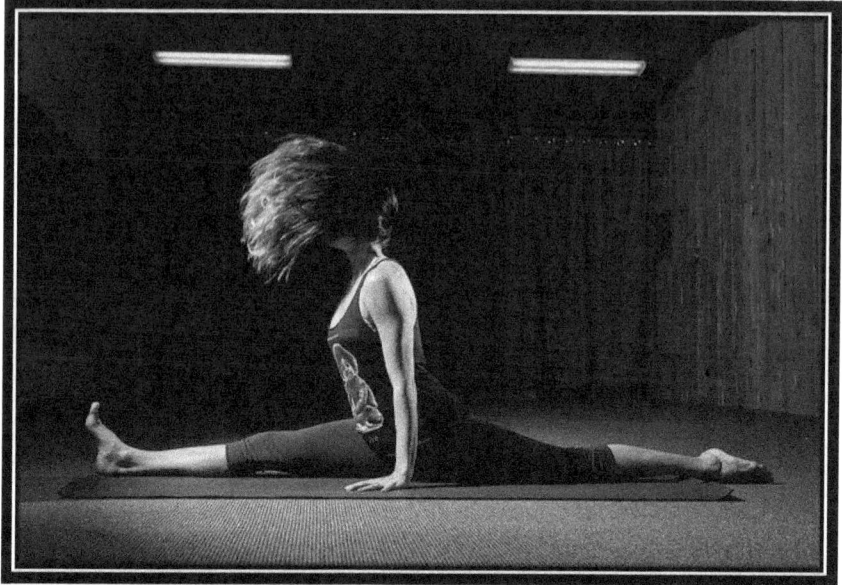

Photo courtesy of a4gpa at Flickr.com

The monkey pose looks easy until you try to get your groin to touch the floor. This pose will strengthen your legs, hips, and help with your sciatica.

1. Start by getting on all fours and step your right foot between your hands.
2. Stretch your left leg out behind you and place the top of your foot onto the floor.
3. Stretch your right leg out in front of you and place the back of your heel on the floor. Keep your arms straight beside you and rest your palms on the floor.
4. Your torso should be straight and your groin should be touching the floor, but go only as far as is comfortable.

5. Hold for five breaths and gently draw your outward-facing leg in, and your inward facing leg in next.
6. Switch sides.

One-Legged King Pidgeon (★★★★★)

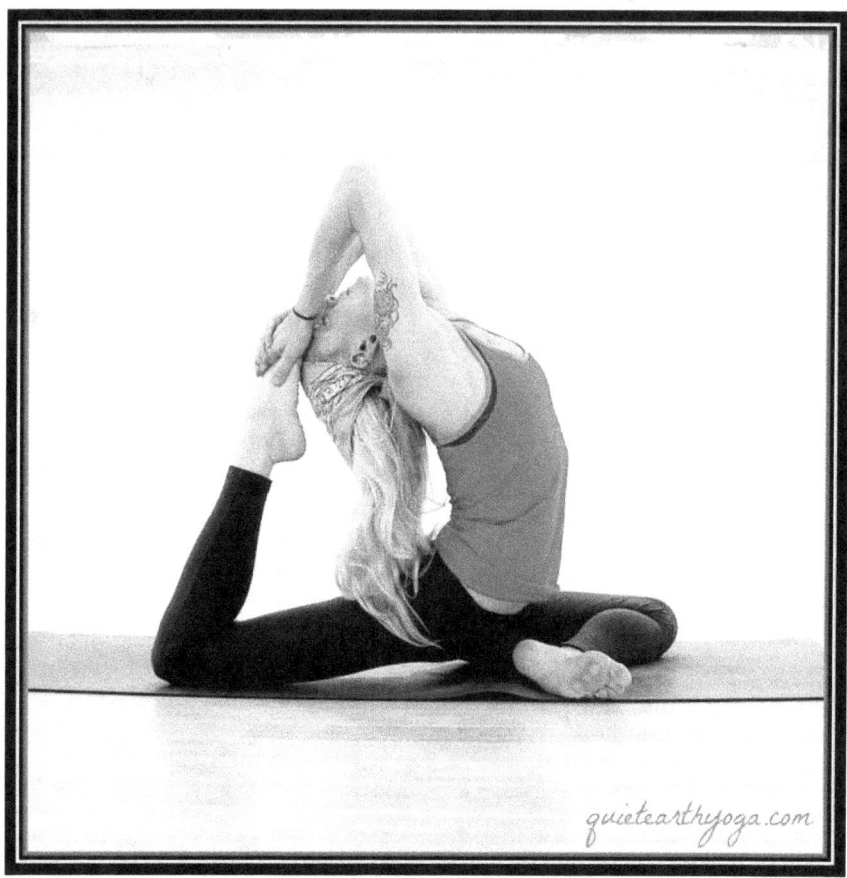

Photo courtesy of Amy at Flickr.com

The one-legged king pigeon looks difficult to perform, but it's still not considered advanced. This is helpful for your thighs, hips, groin, neck, shoulders and spine. If you have a thyroid condition, consider using this pose.

1. Start with the pigeon pose, found <u>here</u>.

2. Sit up tall, firm your abs, and scissor your thighs. Bend your left knee and grab your left foot with your left hand. Bring it up to the back of your head gently.
3. Hold for five breaths and then slowly slide out of the pose.
4. Switch Sides.

Peacock (★★★★☆)

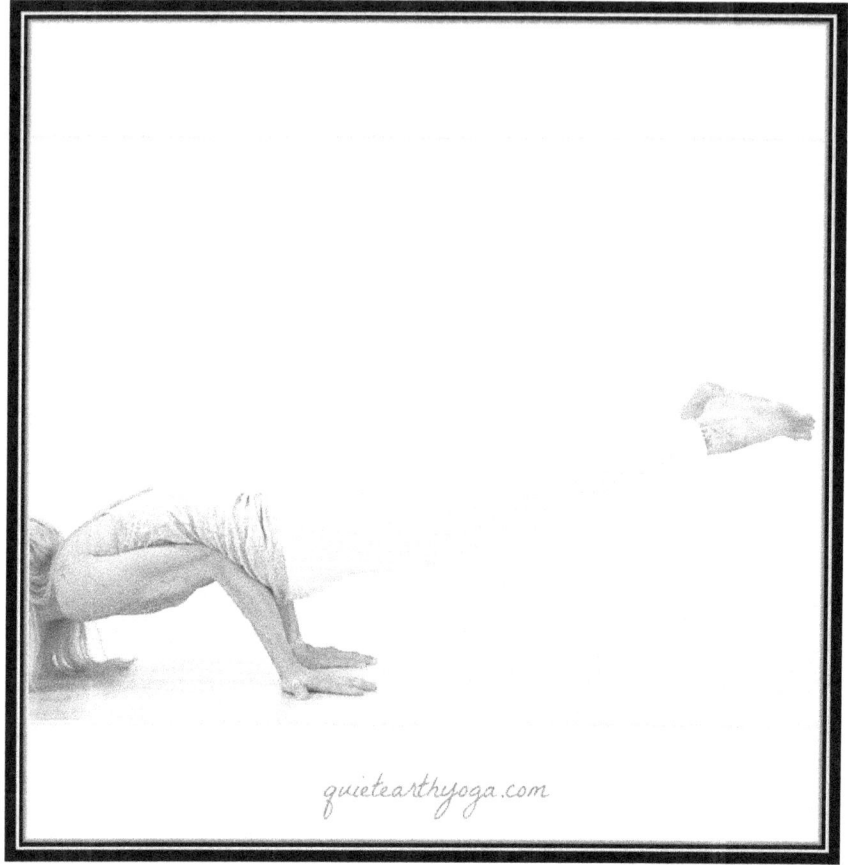

quietearthyoga.com

Photo courtesy of Amy at Flickr.com

The peacock pose will help you strengthen your core, upper body, shoulders, and neck. It's great for relieving stress, depression, and anxiety.

1. Start on all fours and place your hands directly under your shoulders. Your fingertips should be pointing toward you.
2. Straighten your legs behind you and get into the plank position.

3. Now bend your elbows at a ninety-degree angle and gently bring your right leg into the air. Lower our right side onto your right elbow. Do the same with the left side. Keep your legs together and in the air, pointing out behind you.

4. Hold for five breaths and then gently lower to the ground.

Pendant Pose (★★★★☆)

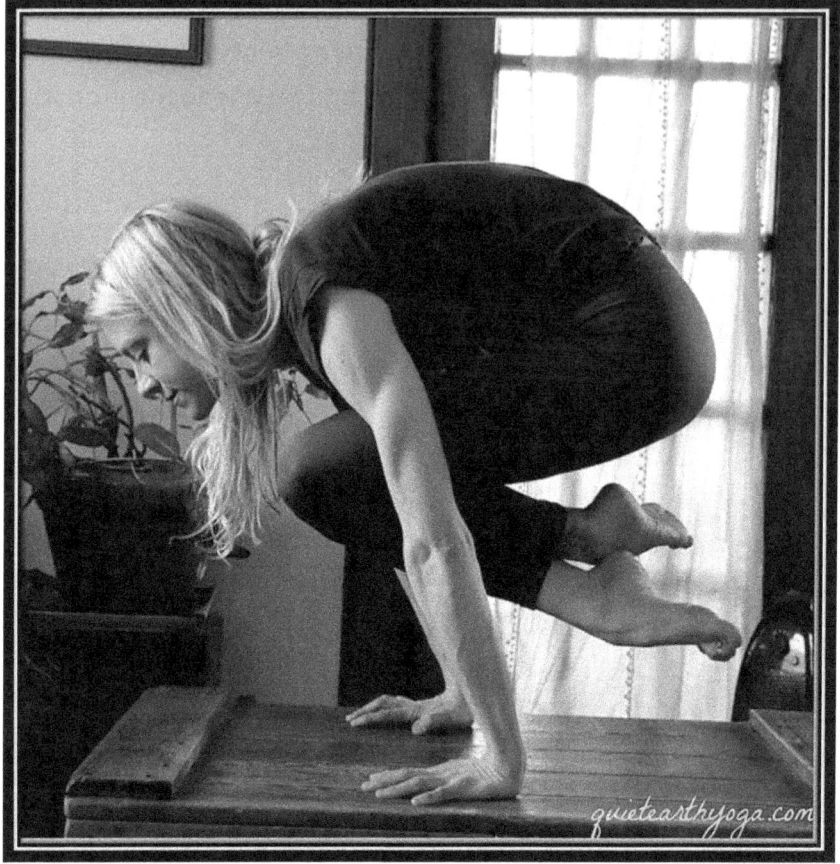

Photo courtesy of Amy at Flickr.com

The pendant pose is an excellent addition to anyone's routine as long as they're able to balance well. It's beneficial for the back, upper body strength, and abs.

1. Start in the cow face pose with your legs crossed and your right knee over your lef.t
2. Then place your palms on the floor at your shoulders and lift your hips off your heels by leaning into your palms.

3. Now look down, lift your hips higher and press firmly into the palms as you lift the feet off the floor.

4. Hold for two or three breaths and then lower back down. Switch sides with your legs and repeat.

Plank (★★☆☆☆)

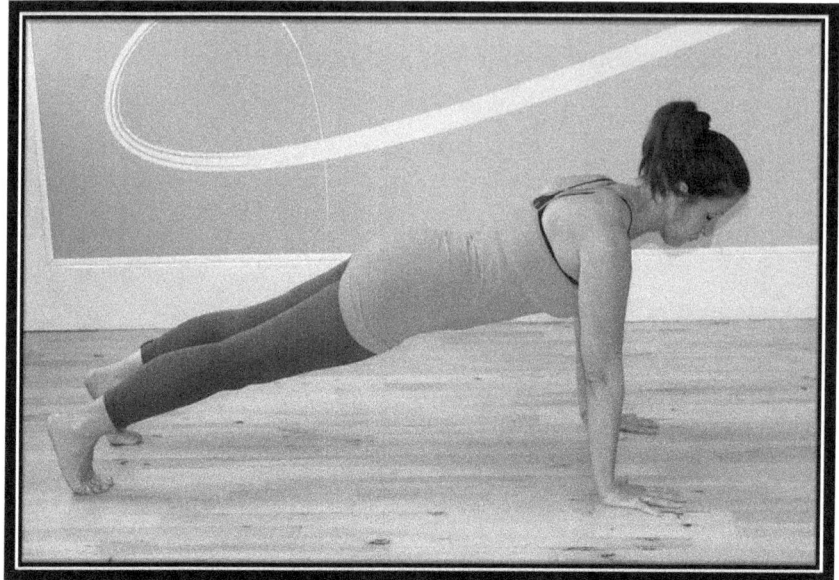

Photo courtesy of yogamama at Flickr.com

The plank is excellent for strengthening your core and your upper arms, as well as lengthening your spine. The pose focuses on helping you strengthen, posture, breathing, and endurance.

1. Begin on all fours with your palms at shoulder width and your knees in line with your hips.
2. Now press into your palms and straighten your legs out behind you, starting with your right and ending with your left. Keep your arms straight and your legs straight.
3. Use your core to keep from moving and hold for five breaths. Gently lower yourself to the ground and rest for two breaths.
4. Come back up into the plank position again, repeat this process three times.

Plow (★★★★☆)

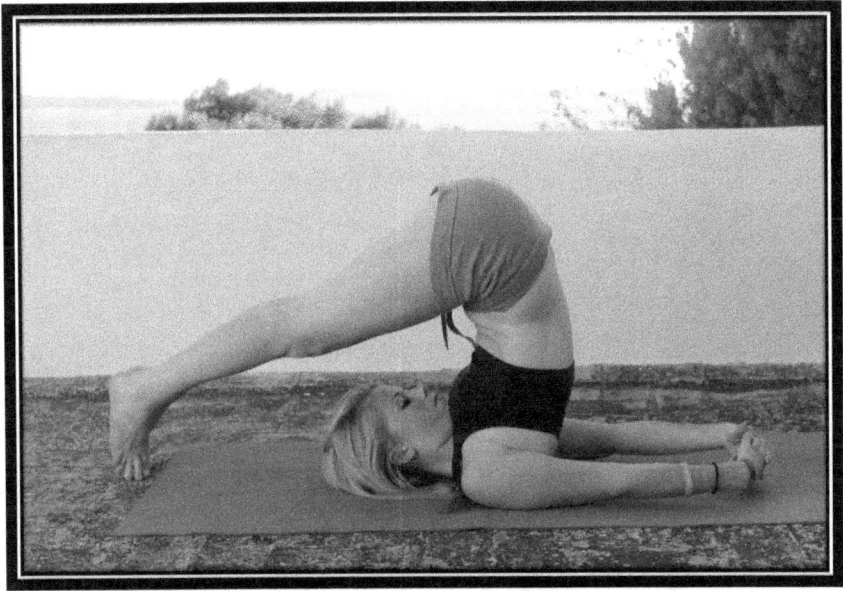

Photo courtesy of yogamama at Flickr.com

The plow will help you stretch your back, neck, hamstrings, shoulders and keep your spine flexible. It's also good for hormonal balance, your thyroid, and insomnia.

1. Lie on your back and keep your knees bent and your feet flat on the floor. Stretch your arms out alongside your body with your palms pressing into the floor.
2. Bring your knees toward your chest and extend your legs over your head. Touch the balls of your feet to the floor behind you.
3. Clasp your hands behind you.
4. Bend your knees and place your right knee next to your right ear and your left knee next to your left ear. Release your

hands and bring them up to rest next to your feet. Hold for five breaths and then release.

Rabbit (★★★★☆)

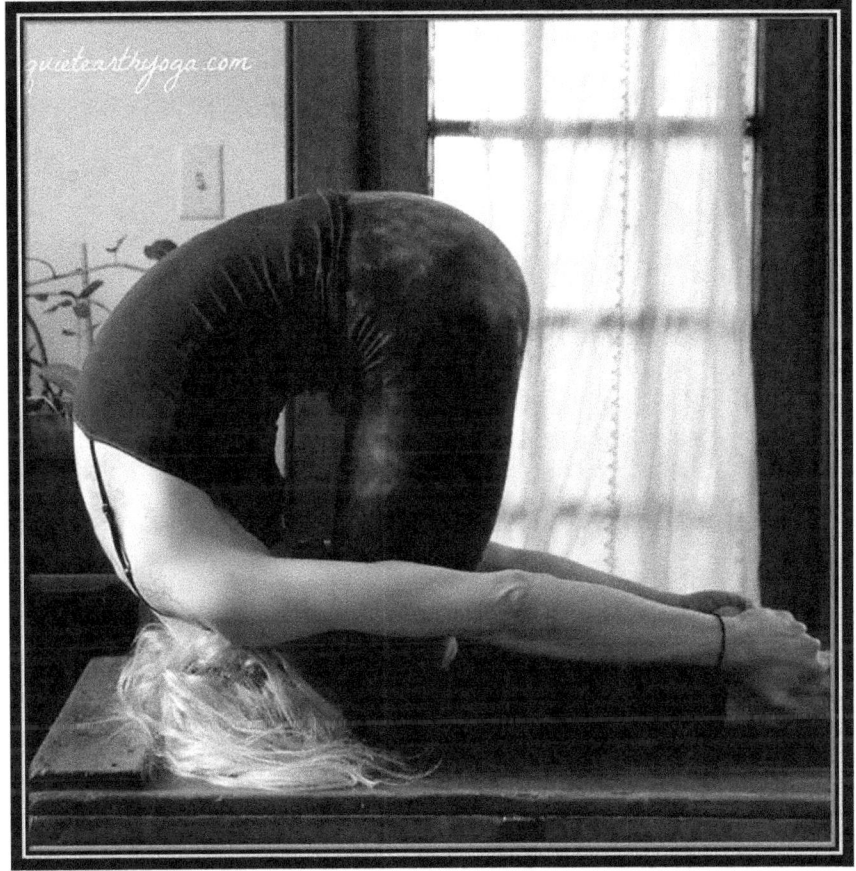

Photo courtesy of Amy at Flickr.com

The rabbit pose will help you stretch your entire body and lengthen your spine. It's also used for headaches, spinal tension, insomnia, neck pain, back pain, and digestion.

1. Start in child's pose and grab the outside edges of your ankles. Roll from your forehead to the crown of your head and inhale and exhale slowly.

2. Extend your arms and shift your body weight forward and onto your head.

3. Reach your arms back so that you're grasping your ankles still and hold this pose for three breaths.

4. Release and relax before you go into the next pose.

Reclining Hero (★☆☆☆☆)

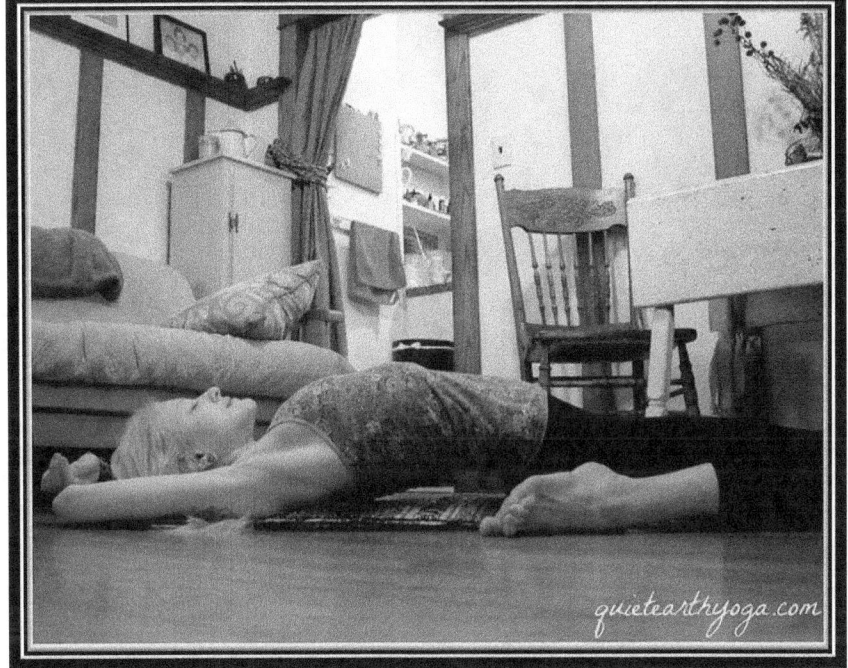

Photo courtesy of Amy at Flickr.com

The reclining hero looks very relaxing, and it is if you're not a beginner. If you're not flexible at this point, do not attempt this pose as it may harm your upper thigh muscles. The reclining hero is used for stretching the tops of your feet, quads, ankles, and abs. It's to help with low energy and fatigue, menstrual pain, and leg flexibility.

1. Start by kneeling on the floor and separating your feet behind you. Lower your butt to the floor between your legs and then slowly slide back.
2. Rest your shoulder blades on the floor behind you and your arms at yours sides with your palms facing up.

3. Breathe deeply for as long as you'd like and then slide your legs forward when you're finished.

Reverse Plank (★★★☆☆)

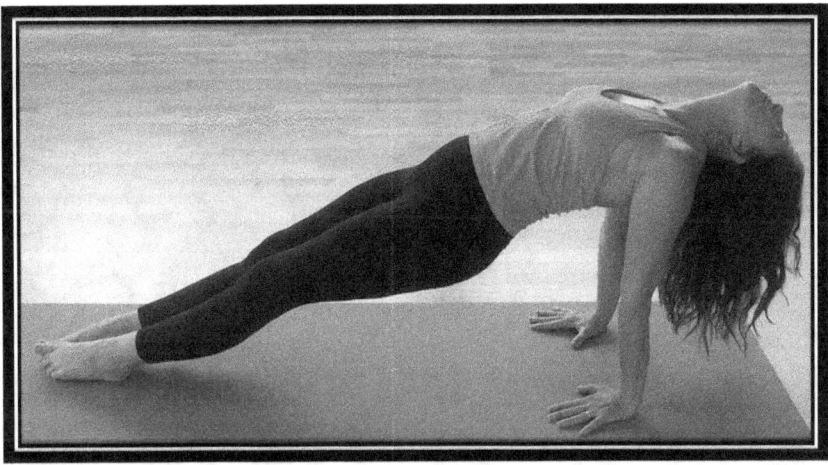

Photo courtesy of yoga mama at Flickr.com

The reverse plank is to strengthen your arms, legs, wrists, and ankles. It also stretches your abs, chest, shoulders, and thighs.

1. Sit straight with your legs out in front of you and your heels touching.
2. Place your hands on the floor in line with your shoulders and your palms facing down. Your fingers should be pointed toward your toes. Now lift your hips until your entire body is straight and your heels are touching the floor.
3. If it's more comfortable, let your head drop back and hold this position for ten deep breaths.
4. Release and repeat five times.

Reverse Warrior (★★★☆☆)

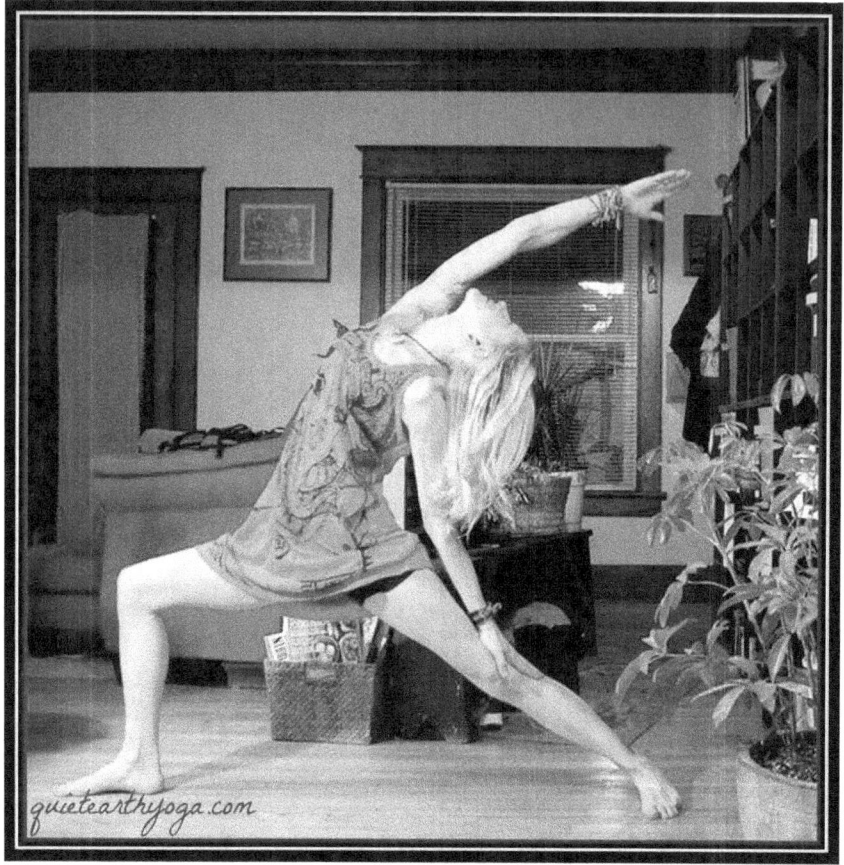

Photo courtesy of Amy at Flickr.com

The reverse warrior looks simple, but having good balance is key here. This is to strengthen your abs, thighs, hips, groin, and keep your spine flexible. Yogis use this pose to ease lower back pain and fatigue.

1. Start in the warrior II pose found here.

2. Now lower your left hand back to your left leg and slide it toward your ankle. Go as far as possible and turn your body to the ceiling. Arch your right arm overhead.
3. This may be as far as you can go, but if you feel comfortable, try to go further.
4. Turn your gaze up and lower your right arm and lift your left arm until they're both at shoulder height.
5. Return to Warrior II pose and then switch sides.

Shoulder Stand (★★★★☆)

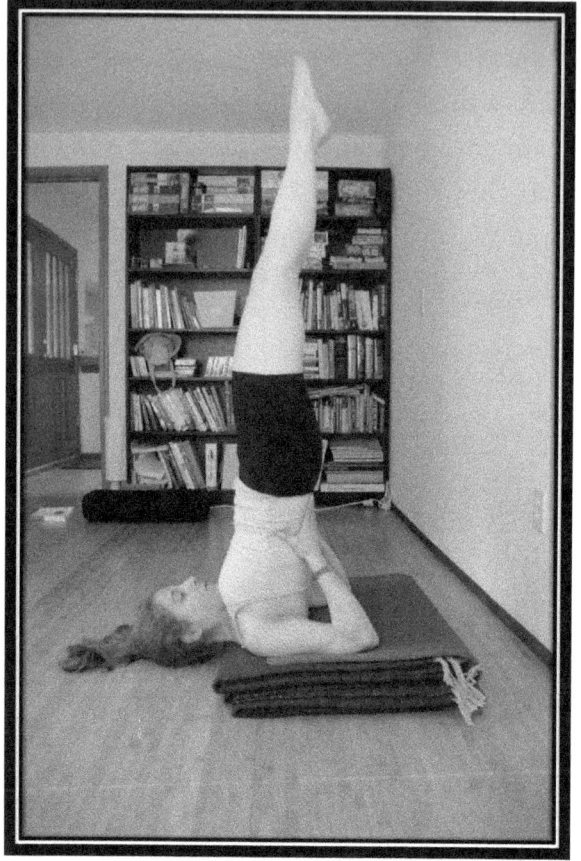

Photo courtesy of Tiffany Berry at Flickr.com

The key to this pose is to stay straight as you're doing it, which is harder than it looks. The pose is excellent for strengthening your upper back, abs, neck, shoulders and arms. It stretches your back and shoulders and helps your circulatory system as well as your thyroid.

1. Lie with your arms at your sides with the palms facing up. You should be on your back. Your feet should be shoulder width apart.
2. While keeping your feet together, raise them off the floor and use your hands on your lower back to support you.
3. Straighten your spine and legs. Breathe deeply and hold the pose for five breaths before sliding out of it like you got into it.

Reference Poses

Warrior Pose II (★☆☆☆☆)

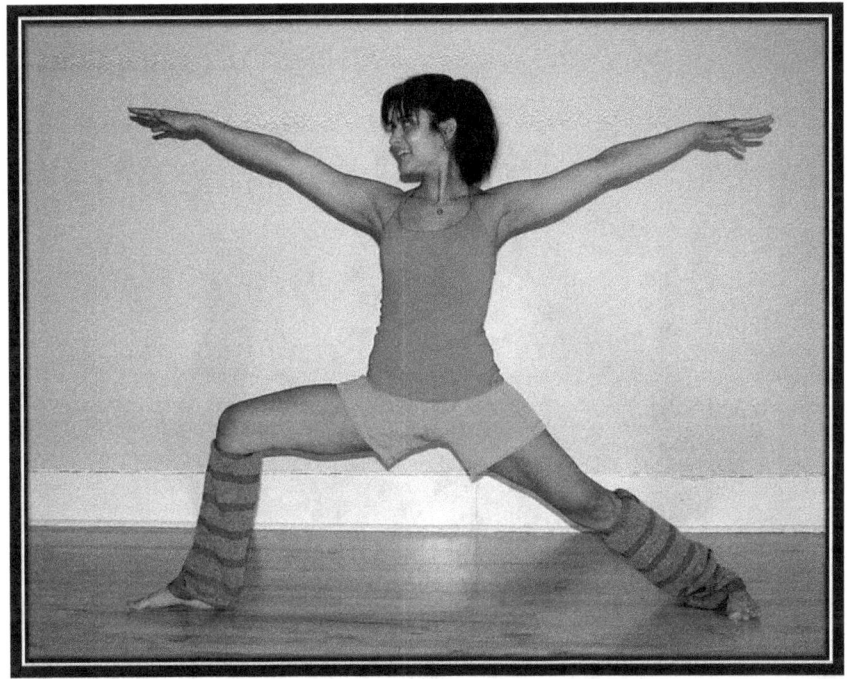

Photo courtesy of Elsie Escobar at Flickr.com

Pigeon Pose (★★★☆☆)

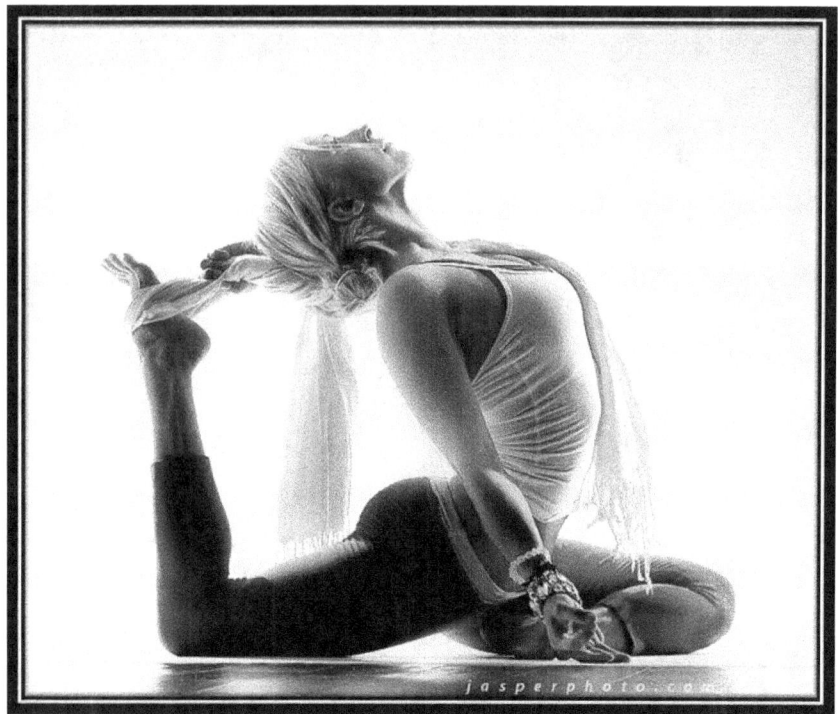

Photo courtesy of Kukhahn Yoga at Flickr.com

Conclusion

Yoga is excellent for your body and your overall health. It helps to lower your stress levels and become in touch with your body and how it's performing. Many people report that after performing yoga for a few weeks, their muscles no longer ache and they're able to sleep better at night. So if you're someone who suffers from muscles and joint aches, insomnia, headaches, abdominal upset, and any other physical or mental ailment, yoga will be good for you.

Remember that while some of these poses look easy to perform, they will put strain on your muscles and your back, so be sure that you've warmed up and you're stretched before you begin. Hydration is also a big part of staying safe and fluid while you're performing yoga, so don't forget to bring a water of bottle.

If you liked this eBook on Yoga Poses, please leave a positive review here. It will only take 1 minute but it is extremely important to me.

Thank you for reading!

With love and respect,

Robert Junior

Some Other Books From Us

Below you can find some of the other books published from us.

★*Preview Start* ★

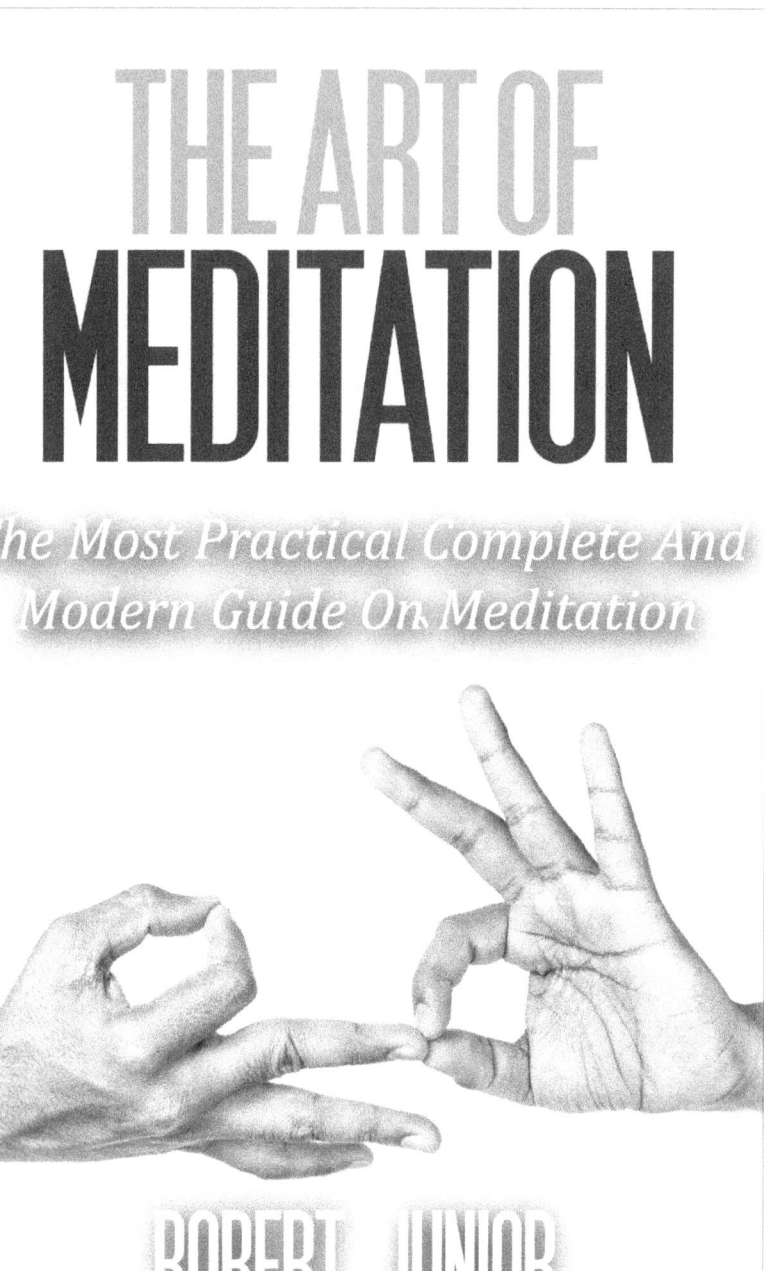

Preface

First of all, let me tell you that you really need to be very happy for downloading my book. *"The Most Practical, Complete And Modern Guide On Meditation: Learn How To Meditate The Easy Proven Way In 24 Hours"*.

This book is in a nutshell the most complete, practical and modern guide a person can read today on meditation. It contains all the steps necessary beautifully combined with lots of pictures and illustrations in order to get you started on the wonderful world of meditation. As you are going to find out by reading this book, through the practice of meditation, you will be able to lower your stress levels, lose weight, become fitter and improve the overall level of your living conditions.

Throughout this book I am going to analyze in great detail many tips and tricks you can use in order not only to get in control of the whole thing but stay in control for the years to come.

As long as you follow the steps and guidelines you will read in this book I can guarantee you that you are going to see the first actual results and feel the difference within weeks.

This book will provide a lot of details on what is meditation, why is it important to practice it, how to be a meditation practitioner, in what aspects of your life you are going to see major improvement and how to stay on track in order to achieve your goals as fast as possible.

Thanks again for downloading this book, I hope you enjoy it!

Table Of Contents

Introduction – History to Meditation

There are techniques of Buddhism, such as meditation, that anyone can adopt.

~ Dalai Lama

Meditation is an ancient practice that is believed to have originated from the Indus Valley. This is where archeologists found wall art that dated back to 3,500 BC depicting people who sat in postures that we would recognize today as meditation postures. Indian scriptures that date back 3,000 years also describe meditation techniques.

Throughout the years after meditation was discovered, religions across the globe adopted various techniques and practices that mimicked meditation. Meditation was introduced to the United States at the same time Yoga was introduced in the early 20th century, and in the '60's there was an explosion of interest in the practice.

Judaism has Hitbodedut and Islam has Tafakkur as well as Sufism. Buddhism uses numerous different forms of meditation, although that's not shocking considering meditation evolved in the Indian region. Even Christianity practices meditation, especially the monks. Monks spend hours inside a room contemplating God daily, which is a form of quiet meditation. Even Catholics use meditation by counting their rosary beads.

So, as you can see, meditation is a worldwide accepted practice of quieting the mind as well as the soul. However, you don't have to be religious in order to believe in and practice the art of meditation. It's simply a tool that will help you relieve your daily stress and help you know yourself better.

Each type of meditation has its unique aspects and should be explored by a person who would like to learn about meditation. You never know if one technique will be better than the other for you if you don't try them. So I encourage you to try out each type a few times before you switch to the next in order to see if it will help you feel calmer and relaxed.

First, let's take a look at the benefits of meditation.

Chapter One – The Benefits of Meditation

Meditation is the practice of achieving a quiet state of mind. There are several different ways to achieve this, which will be discussed in Chapter Two. The more common technique is a sitting position with the legs crossed Lotus style and the hands on the knees. However, there are various different styles and techniques used in meditation such as walking, standing, slow movements, and sitting. For beginners, twenty minutes of meditation daily will help you get into the habit of meditating and help you understand the practice. You can gradually add time to your meditation as you feel more comfortable with it.

So why should you be meditating?

For starters, it's free. Meditation is something you can do anywhere and you can easily practice this on your own with a few guided techniques. It's been proven to be a great short-term stress reliever and a long-term health benefit to those who practice, and the benefits can be felt immediately. However, meditation does take practice and patience.

Compared to other stress-reduction exercises, meditation is one of the better choices because there are no side effects from herbal remedies or prescribed medications. In addition, it's excellent for those who are not able to do strenuous exercises, but it still has some of the benefits of exercise. And the meditation helps us free ourselves from the daily stresses of life without thinking about them.

The first and most prominent benefit to meditation is relaxation. When you are focusing, whether it's on many objects, one object, or on nothing, your mind delves into the theta wave range, which is where your mind is free to think and form thoughts without fear of guilt or shame. In this state, you're more likely to form ideas that are out of the box and your body is more relaxed. Sometimes, people reach this state of mind while they're driving on the highway and can't remember the last five minutes, or while they is brushing their hair in the morning.

Some other psychological benefits to meditation are:

- A boost in happiness by increasing positive emotions, decreasing depression, decreasing anxiety, and decreasing stress.
- Gives you a boost in self-control by helping you regulate emotions and allows you to introspect.
- Improves your productivity by increasing your focus, attention, and ability to multi-task, memory, and ability to be creative.

Meditation is also great for your health. The most common referenced physical benefit is the reduction of stress levels, which affect your health immensely. In fact, most diseases and illnesses that we know of today are actually a secondary illness to stress. Therefore, by reducing your stress levels, you will live a much healthier, vibrant life.

Some other physical benefits of meditation include:

- An increased immune system function.
- Decreased sensitivity to pain.
- Decreased inflammation on the cellular levels.

- Increases the gray matter in your brain.
- Increases the volume of your brain in sections that relate to emotional regulation, positive emotions, and self-control.
- Increases thickness in areas that correspond with focus.
- Lowers your blood pressure while you're meditating and for hours afterward.
- Improves blood flow and circulation throughout your body.
- Lowers your heart rate and respiratory rate.
- Lower your cortisol levels and gives you a feeling of deep relaxation and well-being.

So, as you can see, meditation is an excellent way to make yourself a healthier, happier, better-rounded individual. Remember that you do not have to believe in any type of higher power or being in order to practice meditation, but you can incorporate that into your sessions if you are religious. Either way, meditation is an excellent way to reduce stress levels in your life and get you started on a path to enlightenment and understanding.

★Preview End ★

If you liked the preview you can <u>download a copy of the book here</u>

Free Book

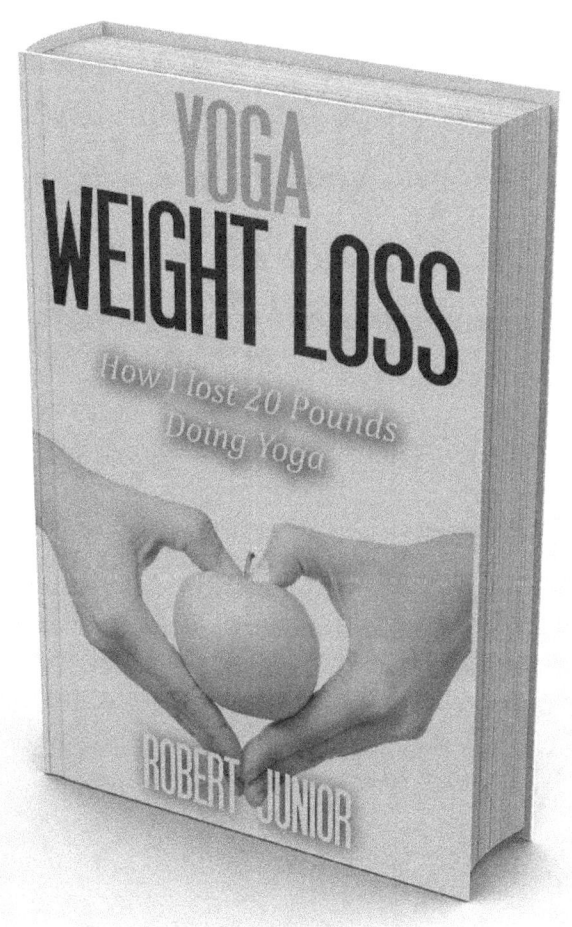

As a Thank you gift for downloading my book, I will give you my new book "Yoga for Weight Loss" for free.

Please follow the link here (http://bit.ly/19eWRoW) to download your free copy of my book "Yoga for Weight Loss" normally sold on Amazon for 2.99$

Thank You